A MOTHER'S 'MEDICAL MAN'

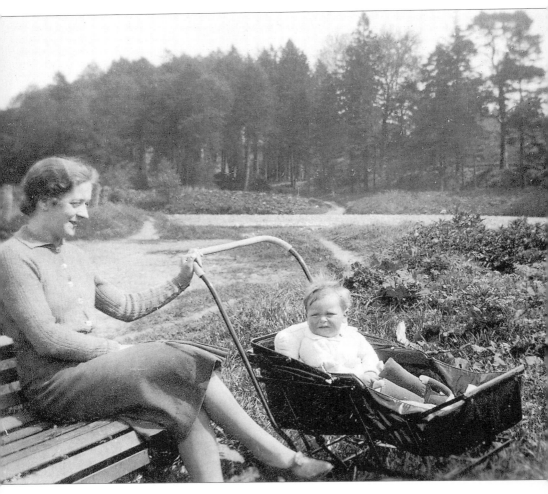

Mother, with me in pram.

A Mother's 'Medical Man'

Ronald G. Wilson

M C

© Ronald G. Wilson, 2002

First published in 2002 by
The Memoir Club
Whitworth Hall
Spennymoor
County Durham

British Library Cataloguing-in-Publication data
A catalogue record for this book is available from the British Library

ISBN 1-84104-055-X

The descriptions of events, incidents and characters featured in this book
are true and correct according to the recollections of the author

Designed and typeset by Carnegie Publishing, Lancaster
Printed in the UK by Bookcraft, Bath

This book is dedicated to two ladies.

The first lady, my mother, struggled incredibly hard to set me on the road to being her 'medical man'. I wish she had lived to see it.

The second lady, Susan my wife, showed me that there was life after a divorce and a heart attack. They never met and I wish they had.

I owe them both a lot!

Contents

List of Illustrations

Foreword

THE following Foreword was written by my mother in about 1963 just prior to her death. It was to be the 'foreword' to a book she had begun to write and on which the first seven chapters of this book are largely based. Her writings remained unknown to me until 1998. They were hand-written in an ordinary exercise book which had lain unopened and unread, among many other memorabilia I have carted round the country, from one house to another, over the years.

'The definition of "Foreword" is given in the *Oxford Dictionary* as: A preface; a short introduction. The story I am about to tell seems to call for just that. It is told by a mother purely and simply for her son and isn't likely to be of any interest to anyone else. Since my "Hero" is a Medical Man there is no need to expatiate on heredity etc., so I will begin my story in the hope that one day he will find time to read it and perhaps find it interesting.'

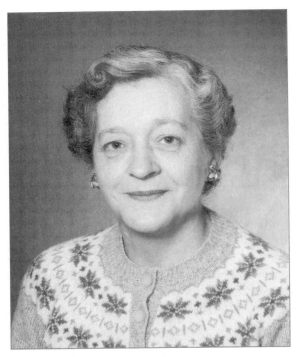

Mother and me at
Graduation.

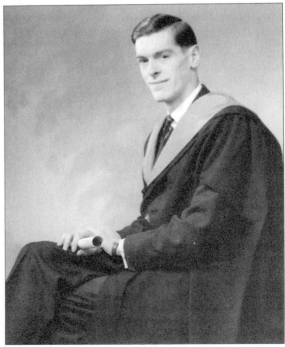

Introduction:
My Parents and Family

MOTHER WAS BORN, prematurely, on Boxing Day 1910. Weighing only 5 lbs, she was not expected to survive. Christened Jeannie (Ena) Watson Cowie Hendry, after her mother who was Isabella Mountain Watson Hendry (née Cowie), her nickname was WC ('Water Closet'). She was not born in Rhodesia House, the family home, as she thought, but in The Cairns Nursing Home, in Blantyre (near Hamilton) close to Glasgow. She had one younger brother, Jim.

Her father, Alexander Wilson Hendry, had been born in Tillycoultry, near Alloa and Stirling. He was a chemist and moved to Blantyre in 1902 and established two shops: one in Blantyre itself and the other in High Blantyre, a short distance south. Mother also qualified as a pharmacist and worked for her father until she got married.

He was a pillar of the local community and served for many years on the local council before becoming a Justice of the Peace in 1933. He has been described as one of 'Nature's Gentlemen' because of his kindness, honesty and humility. Granny Hendry was obviously some-thing of a rebel because of her modern hairstyling and the fact that she smoked cigarettes, unusual for a lady in the 1900s. They were very close and were never heard to argue with each other. They were God-fearing people brought up with a strong sense of duty to God and the Church.

Father was born on 13 November 1903 in the United Free Church Manse in Sandyhills, Shettleston, Glasgow. He was christened Robert Paterson Wilson after his grandfather Robert Semple Wilson. His father, George Lithgow Wilson, was a preacher of the old Calvinistic order who preached of 'The Fear and the Admonition of the Lord'. It was said that his preaching indicated a God of Fear rather than Love. He was a firm believer in Teetotalism and his zeal in enforcing it in the community

1

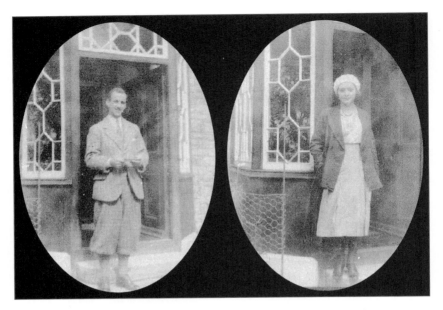

Father and Mother, 1931.

might be viewed, these days, as incitement to riot. A much worst trait was his habit of mocking and patronising his wife who was, in fact, the strength behind the family.

Father's mother was Katherine Burns Wilson (née Paterson). Granny Wilson, as I knew her, married my grandfather on 8 June 1899 in Kelvin, Glasgow: a delightful lady who had had the strength to bear, and rear, six children, three boys and three girls. She was also a child of the manse and was herself one of ten children. All her experience of life, and a big family, was needed to bring up and educate her own six in the face of her husband's personality, some of which regrettably rubbed off on to a number of my father's brothers and sisters.

The family moved to Cullen, on the north-east coast of Scotland, when my father was quite young. He spent all his school years at Fordyce Academy. Father was his mother's favourite and she called him Robin. He was by all accounts, however, a wild child and certainly the wildest of the six of them. He was locked up for the night, by the local policeman, after being caught stealing apples. One of his great-great-great-grand-fathers had been hanged for sheep stealing in Inverness.

In this context it is perhaps important to remember the clan structure in Scotland. The Wilsons are part of the Clan Gunn that hails from the Black Isle, north of Inverness. It was one of the warlike, aggressive, clans. There was a 'black sheep of the family' system in that their names were changed to indicate that they were no longer accepted members of the clan. This is how the names Willson and Patterson came about.

All four grandparents were alive when I was young but only Father's mother lived long enough for me to gain any lasting memory of her. George Lithgow Wilson, his father, who died in 1940, I cannot recall at all. Mother's father died in the early 1940s and her mother in 1944 near Rochdale, Lancashire, where she was living to be near her son, my Uncle Jim, a general practitioner in Shaw.

Father had an Uncle William, a banker who was also an artist. I remember him in his retirement in Milngavie, near Bearsden, in the north-west outskirts of Glasgow. He lived in a small bungalow with a studio in the attic, and a lovely garden. He had an Irish wolfhound, whose name I cannot recall. Nine of his oil paintings of Scottish scenes, and two postcard sized oils, now hang in our house in Spain as a reminder of my Scottish heritage.

Father had a good scholastic record and left Fordyce Academy with Highers in all the usual subjects, and Honours in Latin, German and French. He left Cullen at the age of seventeen and joined the British Linen Bank, at its South Side branch in Glasgow, at the handsome salary of £60 per annum. This post, starting at the bottom of the ladder, had been arranged by his Uncle Willie who was a manager with the British Linen Bank in the city at the time. Father lived with Uncle Willie and his wife, Aunt Agnes, and paid £1 per week for his board.

Banking had not been his own choice; he had wanted to become a vet but this had not been possible as his elder brother Lithgow was studying Medicine in Glasgow. The eldest of the family, 'Telly', was training to be a nurse in Kingston, Surrey. After Father was another daughter named Menie, followed by another Willie who also became a doctor. The youngest of the family, Renee, as was expected of the youngest daughter, stayed at home and looked after her widowed mother.

Mother and Father first met soon after he moved south to Glasgow as her parents were friendly with Willie and Agnes Wilson. Mother was ten years old at the time! I do not know when this young friendship became love but they seem to have been inseparable over many years. Father introduced her to orchestral concerts and light opera, as well as ballroom dancing. He was a fine tenor and sang with the Glasgow Orpheus Choir. They spent most of the holidays camping with their many friends in various parts of Scotland. Father worked, and studied hard, in the bank and gained promotion quite quickly. He moved around all the different departments finishing in the Foreign Department in Glasgow.

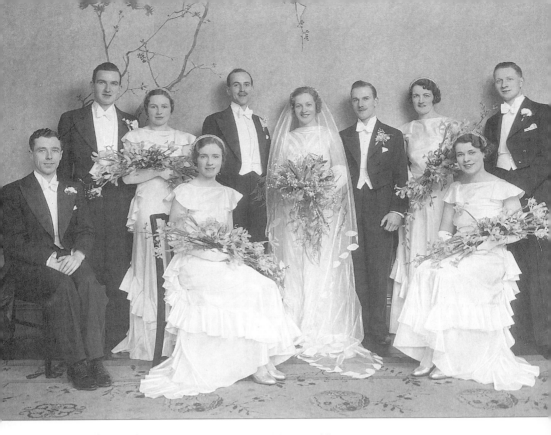

Mother and Father's wedding, 1935.

He had become an experienced after dinner speaker and frequently in demand for this service. A lot of his written material still exists. He also wrote poetry using the pseudonym 'Robin Adair'. I can find no record that any was actually published.

After much discussion with the families they became engaged on 16 March 1932. The three stone diamond ring cost £20 9s. 6d. from Dykes Bros of Glasgow. Sue wears it today and it is as beautiful as ever, although its value is now priceless.

They had to delay the wedding until after her brother, Jim, had finished at Medical School the next summer but as is so often with such plans they were scuppered when he failed his final exams in the June. They had to wait till after October when he passed the resits.

Then the bank took a hand in further delaying their marriage by posting Father to the Foreign Department of the London Office. He had to move almost immediately into digs in 1 Park Road, East Twickenham, and they were apart for over a year.

They were married on 24 April 1935 in Glasgow, the reception being in the Grand Hotel. There were four bridesmaids, Father's three sisters

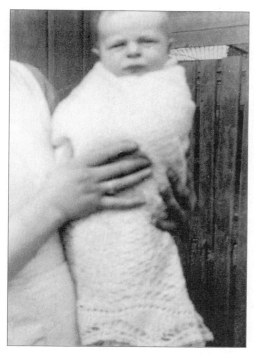

My first photograph?

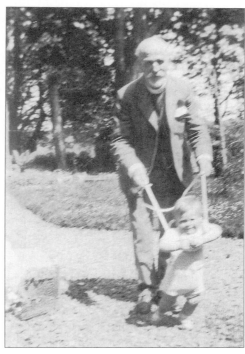

Grandfather Wilson and me,
1938.

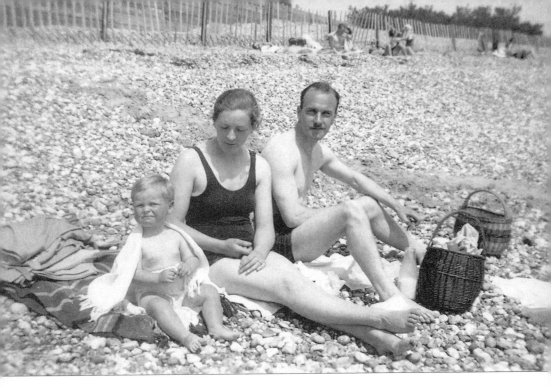

Bognor Regis, 1938.

and Mother's best friend 'Tanna'. Lithgow was the best man and there were three other groomsmen, Father's other two brothers and Mother's brother Jim. I cannot find out where they went on honeymoon.

Their first home was 36 Tudor Drive in Kingston, Surrey, close to the edge of Ham Common. It was a modern semi-detached house that could indeed have been new when they bought it. They called it 'Dalglen'.

In the two years that they lived there, before I was born, they had a lot of friends and a good social life as portrayed in the many photographs of those years that survive. They continued to holiday in Scotland but there was a large contingent of Scottish friends living in those suburbs of London.

Father had made friends with a German couple who lived in Hamburg. They were called Alwin and Louise Mollens and he was, by his uniform, a sea captain. They exchanged lots of letters and photographs between 1934 and 1938 but I cannot find out if either couple visited the other's country. Father certainly was using his German at this stage as a lot of the communications are in German.

Mother went home to Blantyre to have me and I was born in the family home, Rhodesia House, at 11.20 p.m. on 20 April 1937, an Aries by 40 minutes. We returned to Tudor Drive when I was six weeks old.

While I was still too young to remember we moved house, when I was 18 months, to 41 Spencer Road, Strawberry Hill, Twickenham. This was to enable Father to be within walking distance of a station to catch his train to work in the City.

Our first holiday as a family was at Bognor Regis over August Bank Holiday, 1938. There is a collection of photographs of us on the beach. My parents were wearing the swimming costumes of the period and I was evidently able to 'walk'. That year Uncle Jim married Kathleen, a Lancashire lass and a Methodist Minister. The following year my cousin Joyce was born. She eventually had a younger sister, Barbara, by adoption.

A year later in the autumn of 1939 war clouds were gathering and my parents decided to send me back to Blantyre, for safekeeping with Granny Hendry, as everyone firmly believed that London would be bombed as soon as war started. I was by now two and a half and my memory is just able to pick up the threads of the story.

CHAPTER ONE

Earliest Recollections

IT IS A DUBIOUS HONOUR to share the same birth date with Adolf Hitler although, by a happy coincidence, it is also that of my stepson Robbie. At the tender age of two I was of course, at that time, unaware of the connotation.

I was 'evacuated' north to my birthplace on 1 September 1939. One of my parents' friends, Douglas Morrison, was driving north with his best man, Bill Brown, to marry one of my mother's best friends, Betty. The car in which we travelled is my clearest early recollection. Like all cars of that era it was large and black, and was a 1937 Rover Twelve, called 'Big Bertha'.

I have recently discovered a photograph of this car and so I could be accused of jogging my memory. My other clear memories about the same time are of my light blue dressing gown and red pedal car. Although I have black and white photographs of both, none are in colour.

London was not bombed immediately and my parents felt heartbroken that they were separated from me, even though I got on well with Granny and Grandpa Hendry, and their maid Barbara. My parents decided to come north at Christmas and take me back to London with them. I didn't actually recognise my mother, who I had told everyone was in London. I was only convinced that my poor distraught mother was the real one when they produced the red car and the blue dressing gown.

I started to develop one childhood illness after another, some of them more than once. In spite of the belief that you can't have the same one twice I had German measles at least twice. I can remember one of the bouts that was particularly severe for its photophobia and itchy rash, when I was covered in calamine lotion. It is this that I am certain was the cause of my bronchiectasis in later life. To supplement my diet, like most children of those days, I was fed spoonfuls of malt extracts, cod liver oil and concentrated orange juice. In spite of this I was obviously rather a weak child.

I can date these memories reasonably accurately to the age of about two and a half for two reasons. Firstly, after a particularly bad attack of measles I developed osteomyelitis in my right foot, the talus as I subsequently knew. It started with me walking as if I had a fallen arch. In those days there was no such thing as the National Health Service so I was taken to Harley Street where the foot was x-rayed and my whole leg put in plaster. It predated the availability of penicillin, to the populace, by about five years and my parents were told that, even if I overcame the infection, I would be unlikely to be able to walk.

In the light of the continued likelihood of bombing, and my immobility, Mother and I travelled back to Blantyre. I was admitted to the local hospital, Stonehouse, and had the abscess in the bone drained. This has left me with a mark on the dorsum of the right foot that is still visible to this day.

I have no recollection of the operation itself but I was in the hospital for five weeks and clearly remember standing in a cot at a window howling with tears of pain, rage and frustration and hurling my teddy bear out of the window. The teddy bear survived the insult, as I the osteomyelitis and, although I wore a plaster for many months, I was eventually able to walk normally much to the doctors' surprise. Maybe this was when I learnt the caution I applied in later life when giving prognostic opinions to patients. The teddy bear is also a survivor and shares a couch with two colleagues in our present home in Northumberland.

I am confident of the age of these recollections as my own son, James, had his squint operated on, at the age of two, and he has vivid memories of the event. It took another whole year to sort out my foot, in Scotland, with my parents yet again apart. In the meantime Father had moved our furniture and belongings from Spencer Road to 23 Clifden Road, Twickenham.

The London office of the British Linen Bank was housed in Threadneedle Street, at the opposite end to the Bank of England. Father travelled to work daily on the train and he had found that where we lived was still not very convenient for a station and a train service to Waterloo. This, their third house, meant that Father had only a ten-minute walk from Twickenham station and there was a wider selection of both fast and slow trains to town.

This house I can recall vividly. It was a typical 1930s suburban detached house with a large, long, thin garden. It did not have a garage as cars were still a rarity as family owned transport in those days. Telephones were also relatively sparse and we had a standard black bakelite one with a rotating dial. In those days the London telephone numbers were based on the actual name of the postal district. The digits 1 to 9 also carried two or three letters of the alphabet. We were POP 5419.

For such a small family as ours it really was rather a large house. There was a spacious basement and three storeys above ground. The attic rooms were intended for cooks or maids. Quarters like these were still found in the thirties. I have found documents to show that we had not bought this house but rented it at £70 per annum.

The ground floor had a lounge on the left and a dining room to the right of the front door. Behind the dining room was my father's study that had a French window into the garden. In the middle were the stairs up and down. Underneath the up stairs was a toilet and washbasin. Behind the lounge was a large square kitchen in which there was a cylindrical anthracite boiler and rows of kitchen cupboards. Through that towards No. 21 was a scullery and pantry separate from the kitchen: I suspect a design for domestic staff.

There were four bedrooms on the first floor, two small ones at the front, of which I had the one over the dining room, and two larger ones overlooking the garden. My parents used the largest over the kitchen. The all-purpose bathroom was situated between the two back bedrooms. On the top floor there were two rooms at the back with dormer windows overlooking the garden. These were used by us as a storeroom and a playroom for me.

The long garden started with a large lawn, then there was a vegetable patch, a soft fruit area, a number of fruit trees and a compost area. In the event this huge garden was to be a godsend to us during the war. It was divided from the surrounding houses by a six foot solid wooden fence. There was a small front rose-garden with a small central wooden gate. There was no provision for getting a car from the road into the property.

My memory for colours in those early days is very clear. The gate and doors were green and the window frames creamy yellow. The two living room carpets were red, those of the hall and staircase were dark blue, and the kitchen had light blue linoleum. In my father's study he had a large roll-top desk and a wooden swivel chair. This desk had many hidden and secret drawers, and hiding places, and was a great source of amazement and fun for me when I was allowed to play with it. This desk travelled with the family, and then with me, round the country for the next several decades.

There was no central heating in those days and all the rooms had coal fires. One of the cellar rooms was for anthracite and coke, and the other for large lump ordinary coal which would be delivered in huge sacks tipped down a special manhole at the side of the house, in the passage between us and No. 25.

Mrs Smurthwaite, a widow, lived in No. 25. Her house was smaller, and semi-detached with No. 27. It had a glass front porch with some stained glass panels and a stained glass inner door. She did not have a family of her own and she used to spoil me with chocolate biscuits and other treats which were scarce during the war. On the other side, in No. 25, lived a boisterous family but we had little communication, nor I suspect much in common, with them.

I do not remember being at play school, or kindergarten, but Mother took me to endless coffee and afternoon tea visits to friends who also had children.

At the outbreak of war Father had volunteered for the Navy but when they realised he could speak fluent German and Dutch, he was told that he was needed in London. He had instead joined the ARP and as a Warden (well portrayed in *Dad's Army* as Mr Hodges) he would often go back out again, after supper, on his rounds. It was unusual for a man

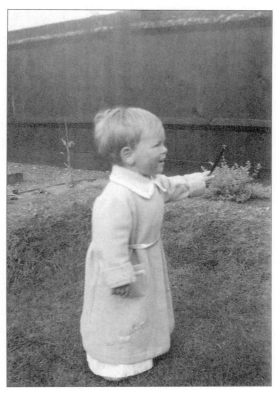

The blue dressing gown.

of his age not to be away at war and apparently still working normally in a bank. This led to some problems for me eventually with bullying at school. I knew nothing of his wartime activities until after it was all over.

Until the bombing raids on London in 1941, I slept upstairs. I caused some consternation when, during a rather rowdy, two table, bridge party, I appeared in my pyjamas and blue dressing gown to complain that I couldn't get to sleep because of 'the bloody noise you're making'.

Later, when the bombing started in earnest, I slept with Mother not in the basement, as you might expect, but under the grand piano in the corner of the lounge between the window and the front hall. Father in his duties saw many people trapped in basements when a house collapsed. This was deemed to permit survival from all but a direct hit. It was certainly much more comfortable than the Anderson shelters that many people had in their gardens.

Two small incendiary bombs penetrated our roof but did not explode and were sticking through the ceiling of one of the attic rooms. Most households were equipped with basic equipment for dealing with such small bombs which were about 18 ins long and 3 ins in diameter. As well as a stirrup pump and a bucket of water there was a long handled scoop with a lid into which these bombs were pushed with a long pole. If the air supply was cut off by the lid they would not burn. In the event Father simply pulled them through the ceiling and removed them to the garden in the scoop. The next day he removed the nose cones, containing the fuses, and emptied out the chemicals. For many years they remained hidden in one of the secret compartments of his desk, a great source of wonderment to me. They disappeared at some stage and I have no idea what happened to them.

The garden had been spared the siting of an air raid shelter and so we were able to maximise the production of fruit and vegetables to expand our diet that was based on the ever decreasing rations that were available from the shops. Left-over greens etc were put to good use when we acquired ten hens, Rhode Island Reds, which, once they were old enough to lay, produced a steady supply of eggs for most of the year. To have eggs when the hens were 'off the lay' we preserved as many as possible in isinglass, a strange liquid which seemed to seal the shells. To do this we had two large clay pots about 2 ft tall that were filled with eggs and this liquid.

I was now over five years of age in 1942 and it was time for me to start school.

CHAPTER TWO

First School

FATHER PLANNED MY EDUCATION almost immediately I was born. He put my name down for Westminster School. Why, I shall never know, in view of all the differences between his deeply Scottish Presbyterian background and the relatively high Church of England influence at Westminster.

This necessitated my going to a preparatory school that was acceptable to Westminster, The Mall School, in Twickenham, a small Prep School of about 150 boys. Mr Ellis was the headmaster, and his wife was the housekeeper/matron. It was a day school but with games on a Wednesday afternoon. We also went to school on Saturday mornings.

The uniform was plain grey short trousers, which was fine if you were not very tall for your age like me, but a little silly if you were twelve and fairly tall. A plain grey blazer, and a matching grey cap, had to be worn at all times outside the school. The tie was red with grey stripes and the school's crest of M S was worn on the cap and the blazer pocket. We were known by the rival schools as 'Mouldy Sausages'.

The school was based on an old Georgian style house which lay in the fork of the road where the two trolleybus services, Numbers 601 and 667, split off from each other. The 601 ran from Twickenham to Kingston and the 667 from Hammersmith Broadway, via Twickenham, to Hampton Court.

I started school in the summer term, May 1942, when I was just turned 5 years of age. I had been taught to read and write by Mother during our prolonged stay in Blantyre the previous year. My form mistress was a Miss MacMahon and there was a grand total of fifteen boys in the class.

During the first three years at the school my parents were sent a small report book where the form teachers commented on my progress and listed my place. I started near the bottom but by the end of my second term had risen to one of the top three places where I stayed for quite a lot of my early time at The Mall.

My second full year at the school began in the autumn of 1943 and the form mistress was Mrs Roake, followed the next summer by Mr Richardson. Now a more usual type of report was produced, by subject, at the end of each term with both a grade given by the relevant teacher and the percentage marks for the end of term test in each subject. Mr Ellis, the Headmaster, then wrote a personal view of the individual's progress, or lack of it, at the end.

My mother took me to school in the very early days but it was not long before I went on the trolleybus on my own. I would frequently walk home to save the fare to spend at the tuck shop that was in the newsagent's next door to the school. In those days no one worried about young children on their own and I never felt threatened in any way. No one ever locked anything away either; I cannot remember coming home to find the front door locked and it was deemed a heinous crime among the boys to steal from one another.

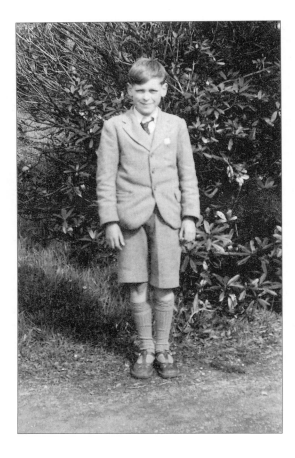

The Mall school uniform, 1947.

Smoking in the bicycle shed, even for the eight year olds, was just as rife in those days as now although I could not see the attraction then or indeed, for cigarette smoking, ever. The majority spent much time, and money, in the tuck shop on frivolities such as pop and ice-lollies. In the 1940s these were home made on the premises and in hot weather quickly ran out. The pop was Tizer made up in glass bottles with the stone cap hinged on wire now found on the trendy bottles of strong beers. The ice-lollies were simple sugary, coloured water frozen in small pots with a tongue depressor as a handle.

The summers then were, seemingly, much hotter than these days. It was a great treat when it became unbearably hot in the classrooms to have the lessons outside in the playing field. We carried the chairs and the blackboard outside and the lesson continued although the distractions were so great I'm not sure how much of the actual lesson we took in.

Mr Summers was the Art master; he was over six feet tall and thin. I remember him as a very pleasant and good teacher. Mr Guild was the Geography master; he was elderly, and indeed retired before I left the Mall. The Maths teacher, whose name escapes me, was somewhat bad tempered, wore a very old three-piece suit and had incredible vision for wrong doing. This would result in a well-aimed piece of chalk striking one on the head or, if he was close enough, a blow with the blackboard rubber to the back of the head. Such behaviour is now banned, of course, but at the time we did not find it unacceptable and neither seemingly did our parents to whom it was little use complaining.

We always had a proper French mistress although to boys of our age the significance of this was lost although we were aware of the attention they would all receive from the male teachers.

We, in spite of the war, were cared for from the nutritional point of view at school. We received a quarter of a pint of milk every day and for lunch we could either take a packed lunch which was eaten in one of the classrooms in the 'annex' building or have the school lunch which could be purchased a term at a time. I varied the lunches partly dependent on our own fruit supply but in the winters I tended to have the cooked one. It was a mixed blessing as there were some good meals and some very bad ones. One did not get the pudding, which tended to be the best bit, unless one had finished the main course. The jam tart and the sago pudding with a spoonful of jam on the top were the prized ones.

We played football in the winter and cricket in the summer, with athletics in addition. My non-abilities with ball games soon became apparent and no position on the games field produced any better results from me than any other. In the end I was usually relegated to being a full back. This would suit me as it meant less rushing about and frequently little to do except cross from one side of the field to the other to try to get between the ball and the goal. Cricket was marginally better although this was more by luck than judgement. I ended up in most games as 12th man so that in most cases the game was won or lost by this stage. If not I tended to shut my eyes and lash out at the ball hard enough to get a boundary if the bat and ball connected. Catching any ball of any size or any shape was, and still is, a matter of luck.

I was marginally better at running track events up to 400 yards. I was lightly built and could accelerate but would soon run out of steam on longer races. I suppose I did not really enjoy sports especially as my poor performance resulted in rude comments from teachers and class-mates alike. This together with the comments about my father being at home began to get to me on occasions and eventually I found myself telling my parents.

This did not have the result that I had expected: i.e. that I would escape the games field on some pretext. Instead Father enrolled me for boxing lessons. A small collapsible ring was erected in one corner of the gym, a place where once again I struggled, weakly and weekly, to climb ropes and jump over wooden horses. We wore very soft boxing gloves and were really, initially at least, simply taught the footwork and various officially recognised punches. Blows if they did land where intended did not tend to inflict pain.

On one memorable occasion I was matched against a boy slightly older than me and a bit bigger. He was also one of those who teased me quite a lot about my games prowess and my father. This he proceeded to do in the ring in front of a number of onlookers. He had a reach longer than mine and was taking a certain amount of delight hitting me quite hard. After one blow to my nose, which brought tears to my eyes, I decided that I had had enough and put all my weight behind a punch, more out of rage than anything else. My blow struck him on the chin as he was trying to retreat out of reach. This accelerated his backwards pace and he fell over the ropes, out of the ring and struck the back of his head on the radiator on the wall as he went down.

He was out cold for a short time and of course I thought that I had killed him. He came round fairly quickly and evidently lacking any serious or permanent damage. I did not enter that boxing ring, or any other for that matter, again although much to my surprise and long lasting education he was never rude to me again.

The whole class would go to the outdoor swimming baths in

Twickenham, down by the river in the centre of the town. We were encouraged to try all the classical front and back strokes as well as rudimentary diving techniques. Although I enjoyed these trips I never felt that swimming was going to be a hobby of mine and this was reinforced by two events.

The first was that I invariably got an ear infection after visits to the baths and these could be very painful. Only Sulfonamides were available in those days and they were terrible to try to swallow. The large tablets had to be crushed and mixed with our home-made strawberry or raspberry jam before I could get them down. As a result of one of these infections with excruciating, throbbing, pain the pain suddenly disappeared and a lot of pus came out of the ear. The drum had perforated and of course I was deaf on that side for quite a long time. It also meant that I couldn't swim even if I'd wanted to.

The second event was during a visit to Kew Gardens when I was pushed into one of the duck ponds by a 'friend' and had a severe panicking session as I tried to get out again. A lot of water went in my ears again but worse was the amount I swallowed before I was on dry land. After that I never swam for pleasure, only for necessity.

It was during one of our school trips to the baths that an incident happened that was to have severe repercussions at school. On this trip the Welsh Maths master accompanied us and a little to my surprise insisted on coming into the changing room while we dried off and changed back into school uniform. He went further in helping some of us to dry ourselves 'properly' meaning the bit between our legs.

I, and at least one other boy, told our parents about this that evening and asked if this was normal activity for a schoolmaster. My parents, I remember, were very calm considering the outrage at paedophilia today and simply told me that I had been right to tell them immediately. That night, when he went out after supper, my father did not go on his ARP rounds but to the school to appraise the headmaster of the morning's happenings. Being innocents we were all a little puzzled to discover that the following morning the school had a vacancy for a Maths teacher.

Father continued to try to get me interested, and involved, in some form of sports activity. Twickenham Rugby Football ground was just the other side of the railway station and he took me there one day when there was a trial for the Junior Harlequins. The oval shape of the ball made it even less likely that I could handle it. I wasn't invited to join. I did, however, find it a more enjoyable game to watch than football, and so started to go to the games on a Saturday afternoon.

There were two parents' sports days at The Mall, one in the summer where there were the usual silly races such as the three-legged, sack and the egg and spoon. Father was rather good at these although I was somewhat embarrassed by his efforts. In the winter there was a football match between the school's first eleven and a parents' side. Father was quite good with a football but thoroughly embarrassed me on one occasion by turning up to play in a borrowed Wasps' rugby strip.

A sport that he introduced me to, and which I did become interested and involved in then and in later years, was rowing. On Eel Pie Island, which lies in the middle of the Thames in the centre of Twickenham, there was a rowing club. It had a static tank in which you could learn and practise rowing techniques before venturing on to the water. As the seats were on *terra firma*, and not on a boat, the blades of the oars had slits in them to let the water through. I expect there are others in the country but I have never come across another one.

I found that coxed pairs and fours were good fun as these were quite sturdy Thames rowing boats rather than the long narrow racing boats used as sculls and eights. They were very safe and we youngsters could learn all that was needed for later racing in them.

A sport which was not an approved one but one which a lot of us participated in was jumping off trolleybuses at the junction where the two routes separated. The reason for the development of the sport was that the 667 stopped outside the school but the 601 went round the back and there was not a stop for a few hundred yards. If on the 601, one jumped off as it turned left. There was a certain skill required as the driver slowed down to let the trolley arms take the points without coming off and then accelerated quickly round the bend. You couldn't see the contact point of the trolley arm with the wires from the platform so the skill was in judging the position of the whole bus relative to the points.

There were accidents and a few grazed knees but as one was jumping away from the traffic there was little danger of severe injury. It was eventually banned as a sport by the school but this did little to deter the enthusiasts until one day a trolley arm came off its wire just as I was leaving the platform. Only those who remember trolleybuses will know that the effect of the letting loose of the spring of one arm can bounce the other arm off as well with the result that the whole trolleybus jumps. I was thrown unceremoniously in a wide arc through the air to land heavily half on the pavement and half against the wall. Luckily, apart from grazed hands, elbows and knees only my pride was hurt but it did deter me from that sport for some time.

My only bad memories of The Mall were the times when I was 'kept in' after school, mainly for non-doing of homework but also occasionally for some misdemeanour in the eyes of the teachers. The remaining at school was not too bad. The wrath of my father was far worse.

Looking back it is interesting to remember that all the time I was 'enjoying' myself at school there was a war raging around me of which I was becoming more and more aware as I got older.

CHAPTER THREE

Memories of the War

F ATHER SERVED in the ARP, as the warden service was known, from
3 September 1939 until 1 July 1945, although he did an anti-gas course
in the City earlier than that. He was called up in September 1942 and
was accepted by Navy Board 2 in Kingston on the 23rd, and classified
medically grade 1 on the 29th. In the event he stayed in his post at the
bank because of his language skills.

My memories of the war are based on sights and sounds. The obsession
with the blackout, which was one of the jobs my father had to enforce
as an Air Raid Precaution warden, and the crisscross tape on the windows
to lessen the fragmentation by bomb blast, are two vivid memories.

The sounds that stick most were the air-raid sirens. There were two
separate sounds. The first was the 'alert' which was a fluctuating up and
down wailing noise at which everyone stopped what they were doing
and looked for the nearest shelter. The second was the 'all clear', a long
single sound that died away slowly. Long after the war had finished any
such a noise from a factory would turn my blood cold.

Other sounds were the different engine noises of the British and
German aircraft. The British always had a very smooth sound. I can
still detect the sound of these engines today at a good distance indicating
a Spitfire or possibly the bigger Lancaster. German aircraft had very
rough running engines due to the fact that many had diesel engines. In
the event it meant that most people could determine the nationality,
and therefore the risk, from an approaching plane long before they could
see it.

Our new house in Clifden Road was only separated from the railway
line by a large girls' school that the Germans believed was a large factory.
During the heavy raids of 1941 and 1942 they frequently dropped bombs
on the area. The following morning there was always a lot of metal
fragments, shrapnel, lying around in the streets and one quickly realised
why a tin helmet had to be worn at night. The anti aircraft guns and

the searchlights were constantly moved around and quite often there would be one or the other parked in the station yard when I would go along in the evenings to meet Father.

After a night of ARP patrol he would come home and tell us frightening tales of destruction: houses that had been totally flattened and others in which all the occupants had been killed by the blast of a bomb but the house looked undamaged except there was no glass in the windows and the front and back doors had changed places, somehow passing each other on the way.

He himself received a slight injury when he was moving an unexploded incendiary bomb which went off as he was picking it up in the scoop. The flare of the phosphorus just caught the instep of one foot and burnt it through his boots. It healed but he was left with very rough and discoloured skin.

I was fascinated by the barrage balloons that were to be found in the parks and open spaces around Twickenham and neighbouring Richmond. They reminded me of Dumbo's mother in the cartoon that, in those days, was new.

One day the whole school had been sent down to the shelters at the end of the playing fields. It was lunchtime, and the class prefects were sent up to collect the lunch. I was on my second trip up to the school, a distance of about 150–200 yards, and was returning with a tray of jam tart. I paused at the corner of the gym and peeped round to see if the coast was clear before making the dash to the shelter. All seeming clear, I set off to run as fast as I could but after a few paces I heard the unmistakable sound of the engines of a German plane.

I did a swift reversal, of course, back towards the gym when over the playing field going in the opposite direction, at tree top height, flew an Me 110 which proceeded to machine-gun the back straight of the school's running track on the other side of the playing field. So far the tray of jam tart had remained intact but as I skidded back round the corner of the gym my feet went from under me, and the tray landed in the dust. After recovering my composure I ran carefully down to the shelter where we tried, unsuccessfully, to scrape the dust off the surface of the jam.

My best friend at school was Alistair Conn. Surprisingly his birthday was also 20 April but he was half an hour older than me (or was it the other way round?). It was quite a coincidence though, particularly to be in the same class. He lived in Radnor Road that was on one of the routes that I could take home, and I often stopped at his house. Mother was always telephoned in those cases to let her know where I was and that I would, possibly, be staying for tea. His father worked at the

Teddington Hydrographic Tank and was involved in the testing of Barnes Wallis's bouncing bomb.

To get from his house to ours I had to go through a narrow lane between Radnor Road and Pope's Grove. On one occasion the road was cordoned off with the sign indicating that there was an unexploded bomb in the vicinity. It turned out to be in the garden on the right hand side of the lane and a shaft had to be dug down to reach it. I was told by my parents not to go there again until the bomb had been removed. I, of course, went back every day to see what progress had been made.

I learned a lot from that experience – that the explosive was steamed out after the fuse or fuses had been removed or, in the case of trembler delayed action fuses, by pouring in a gelatinous substance to stop the mechanism. I also learned that bombs arm themselves after falling for so long through the air and if dropped at low level they wouldn't arm. The Argentinians forgot some of this general knowledge in the Falklands war.

When the bomb was deemed safe to move it was hoisted out of the hole. I remember seeing it dangling from the tripod that had been erected over the hole and thinking that it was rather large and if it had gone off how much damage it would have done to the surrounding houses. It turned out that it was one of the largest actual bombs that the Germans dropped on London; I believe it weighed 1000 kilograms.

The other bomb that I recall seeing was even bigger and more dangerous in that it was what was called an aerial mine. It looked like a dustbin and it was dangling from a parachute which was caught in a tree on the edge of Strawberry Hill golf course. Only later did it dawn on me then that it had landed close to my father's ARP post, a small hut on the golf course, only a few yards away.

A sound that no one will ever forget was the V1, pilotless, flying bomb. Its engine was a ramjet that emitted a curious burring/buzzing noise, hence the nickname 'Buzz Bombs'. They were aimed in the general direction of London and where they landed depended firstly on the expenditure of their fuel, and secondly what the bomb did when the engine cut out. The ominous sign for those on the ground either watching it or simply hearing one was the utter silence when that engine cut out. Thereafter there was no knowing if it would go on gliding and descend slowly, landing up to miles further on, or whether it would nose dive vertically into the ground.

They were very indiscriminate and destructive. I began to wonder if they were out to get my father as three of them landed on the golf course round his ARP hut and each time the clock was knocked off the wall. After the third time they decided to leave it on the floor in case the next one broke it. I was able to realise by this stage that there was this rather strange sense of humour about.

Much worse were the V2s. They carried twice as much explosive and arrived totally without warning. The only one that actually landed near us hit a crowded pub, down near the river at Grotto Road, and the death toll was high. The whole area where the pub had been was just a flat area of rubble. I had heard the explosion, which was obviously quite near, and when I went down on to the main road in the morning there was not a single pane of plate glass left intact in the shops all along the street and it was inches thick on the pavements.

The population was just going about its business, walking over it carefully, while the shopkeepers did their best to cope. It was quite amazing how quickly it seemed that everything got cleared up, as if they were setting a challenge to see what was going to happen next. Everyone knew, by this time, that the end of the war was just a matter of time but they were getting very tired of it and wondering, after all that they had been through, whether they would live to see peace again.

The thing I remember most vividly about the war's end was the VE parade in London. Father took Mother and me up to town which of course was a great excitement for me as I was now nine. We watched the parade from his office on the second floor overlooking Threadneedle Street. There were huge crowds bulging from the pavement into the road with a line of servicemen every few yards between them and the parade that seemed to go on for ever.

Among the photographs which I have recently found are two of that office. At the time I thought how spartan it was with large expanses of bare desks and lots of telephones. All I knew was that it was the foreign department of the bank but up till that moment had not really thought what a foreign department that needed German and Dutch speakers could possibly do during the war.

CHAPTER FOUR

The Dutch Connection

THROUGHOUT THE WAR we had a regular visitor to the house who would come home with my father on a Friday night and return to town with him on Monday morning. I knew him as Uncle Jo. He was a Dutchman and always brought me a present when he came to see us. He was a typical Dutchman in that he was well built but rotund, had a rather wide neck and a large, almost bald, head. He smoked cigars whereas my father smoked Capstan Full Strength or Kensitas. Mother smoked Players No. 1 or Passing Clouds, which were not round but oval.

Joseph Wondergem (pronounced Vonderchem) was his full name. When with us he would work in the garden, which I am sure was a great help to my father. Most memorably I recall an occasion when one of the hens got a large stone stuck in her crop. They all had individual names and the thought of losing one upset everyone in the family. This particular one was called Henrietta. An operation was deemed necessary so she was placed on the kitchen table, fed some drops of alcohol, and held firmly down by all of us except Uncle Jo who made a cut in the crop with a sharp penknife and removed the stone. Henrietta, once over her hangover, lived to a ripe old age as no one could bring themselves to even thinking about eating her.

The only other thing that I knew about Uncle Jo, at this time, was that his wife, Nell, was still in occupied Holland. He rarely spoke about this, was extremely worried about her safety and did not get any messages from Holland about how she was. After the war I got to hear the story of how he and my father came to be close.

At the outbreak of war he had been Sergeant Wondergem of the Royal Netherlands' Mounted Police. He was, at some stage as the Germans invaded Holland, assigned to protect the Royal Household and was involved in the evacuation of the Queen from Holland, under the eyes of the advancing Germans, by a British destroyer. Once in England

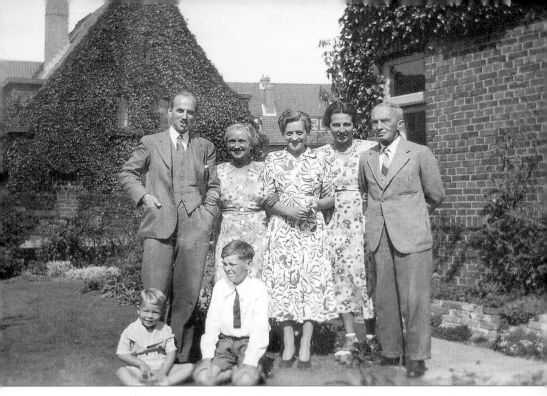

Dutch connections, 1949.

he, being now close to the Royal household, was picked to help run the government in exile through the duration of the war.

It was realised that the Dutch servicemen and women who had escaped captivity, whether it was in Europe or in the Far East, would need some form of financial institution to protect not only the Government's monies but also for their day to day banking needs. Uncle Jo was given the task of establishing such an institution. Someone in the banking circle knew that Father was fluent in Dutch so it was suggested that he came to see Father to discuss the proposal.

The Dutch Bank (in exile) was established and by the end of the war was quite a large organisation. I recall my father explaining to me that for all the millions of Dutch guilders that had passed through the bank up to the time it was shut down and the responsibility returned to the true Bank in Holland, the police sergeant turned banker had only lost something like the equivalent of £5.

My only indication as to any high level of the Dutch Government involvement is a letter dated 16 October 1943 from the 'Netherlands Secretary of State for General and Home Affairs' inviting Father to dinner at his official residence.

I was unaware of the significance of where in Holland Aunty Nellie, as I came to call her, was living. I knew she lived near Arnhem; but even more worrying for Uncle Jo, she actually lived in Oosterbeck. It was only after Holland was liberated that we learned that she was safe. It was much later before we heard what she herself had been up to during the battle, and it was not till I visited Oosterbeck many years later that I found that their house was very close to the church on the river where the paratroopers made their last stand.

At the time of the invasion of Holland Nellie had hidden all her good linen inside the furniture of the house, mainly underneath the dining room tabletop. During the battle she had brought them out and torn them all up into bandages for the injured. She had trained as a nurse and her house had become a field dressing station. Apparently at one stage the house was absolutely crammed with wounded soldiers. She was lucky in the event not to have suffered from reprisal activity by the Germans; as it was the inhabitants of Arnhem and Oosterbeck had a very unpleasant time until the liberation.

At the end of the war Uncle Jo returned to Holland with the rest of what was the Dutch Government in exile. He, not surprisingly in view of the work he had done in London, was rewarded with a post in the Ministry of Welfare.

One of the biggest problems he faced was the plight of the many refugee children left orphaned as a result of the war. It was suggested that some came to Britain to stay with the families who had helped the Dutch Government in exile. Mother and Father agreed to take one of the first in 1945. His name was Yoppi Schut and he was a really difficult problem for my parents to cope with. Being used to simply staying alive he still had the habits required to do this in war-torn Holland and had a habit of stealing. Nothing my parents seemed to do would stop it.

At the end of his stay Mother said she would not have another orphan to stay in the light of our experience. This upset Uncle Jo who had not intended such an outcome especially with such close friends. Yoppi did not view the experience in the same light as ourselves and much to our surprise out of the blue came a typical Dutch, hand decorated, tile plaque with thanks to us for having him for the year. I always wondered what became of him.

Our next contact with Uncle Jo was to learn that Auntie Nellie was pregnant and nine months later they had a boy whom they christened Robbie, after my father.

In the spring of 1949, when Holland was more back to normal and young Robbie was a toddler, all of us were invited over to Holland.

I was approaching the eleven plus stage and because of the dates that my father and Uncle Jo could both get time off work together, it meant that I would have to be taken out of school in May for two weeks. Mr Ellis refused to give permission for this, partly because of the impending exam but also he argued that I had had so much time off school over the years, up to 52 days in one term and 30 days in two others, due to my chronic ill health, any more was unjustified.

My father went to the school to discuss it but Mr Ellis was adamant. My father was just as adamant that I was going to Holland and that it would be good educational value for me. In the end a vague threat of expulsion if I went was made. I went and wasn't expelled.

We flew from Heathrow in a Convair 340 of the Dutch airline KLM. This plane is a twin radial-engined plane roughly the size of a Dakota but was specifically built as a civilian one. It was also new in that it had a tricycle undercarriage, and not a tail wheel. This meant that the floor of the plane was level and not sloping up from the back to the front.

To keep his word about my education I remember Father trailed us round all the important art galleries, museums and historical sights in Holland. The first time I saw the airborne cemetery at Arnhem I wasn't really prepared for the number of headstones: row upon row with so many inscribed 'Known only to God'.

I cannot recall that Father and Uncle Jo ever saw one another again although they regularly wrote to each other. Jo died in 1989 when he would have been about eighty-five. We continued to swap Christmas and birthday cards until Auntie Nellie died in 1998.

CHAPTER FIVE

The Post-War Years in London, 1945–1949

T HE END OF THE WAR brought with it an incredibly different way of life. It must have been a return to something like normality for the adults but for those of us who had no real recollections of any other way of life there was a sudden freedom. It was a novelty for there to be lights on in the streets after dark. Signposts, which had all been removed to try to confuse the Germans if they had succeeded in invading, were replaced.

Rationing, which we had all endured throughout the war, was not lifted for many years and in some respects got worse in the first few post-war years. We did, however, see some of the foods and fruit that I only knew by name: peaches and bananas for instance. Young as I was, I found it strange that after Winston Churchill had steered the country through to win the war he was resoundingly defeated in the early post-war election. This coupled with the continued shortages and the insistence on nationalisation of everything to produce a seemingly poorer service for years to come probably set my political stance for life.

In those days we spent a lot of time visiting the sights of London that my parents had known before the war and which I had not seen. Now nine years of age, I was taken to see shops like Dickens and Jones, Harrods and Selfridges. The shop nearer home, which I can recall very well, was Bentalls in Kingston where Mother and Father would go to the afternoon tea dances. My main interest in those outings was listening to the bands, and orchestras, and it is here that I must have acquired my interest in rhythm and big band music.

Kingston and Hampton Court were places that I soon started to go to on my own because of the direct trolleybus services from Twickenham. In the opposite direction, downstream on the Thames, was Richmond. It was a beautiful walk along the towpath and it was possible to use the

London Transport 90 bus service to go one way or the other. Going in the direction of town the 667 trolleybus would take me to Hammersmith Broadway, or Brentford for variety. The greatest adventure, however, in those days was to take the 90B through Hounslow to Heathrow Airport.

The first time I ever went there were only a few Nissen huts and some tents. These were quickly replaced by long, low two-storey buildings alongside the road (Bath Road) and it was exciting to see all the new names of airlines and freight companies which had been added between visits.

In the latter days at The Mall, after the war had finished, I cycled to school and this of course opened out an entire new dimension in my ability to explore the locality, particularly in the summer. I would cycle to Heathrow taking a picnic once Terminal 1 was built, with its roof viewing terrace. It is amazing to remember those days now when there are four Terminals and a fifth one about to be built. All the open space that used to exist around the runways has been swallowed up with buildings.

Apart from the buses and trolleybuses there were two other ways to get to town and they were by the Southern Region trains to Waterloo and by the Underground, District Line. It is remarkable that in the 20s and 30s the development of the suburbs of London should have brought along the development of a very farsighted transport system based on eco-friendly electric traction.

I often cycled round to the station to meet Father and it was on one of these occasions that I attained my second scar that remains with me today. The local council used a quick and cheap way of resurfacing their roads by spraying tar on the surface and then sprinkling fine yellow gravel on top. The station yard had just been done this way and as I arrived, too fast, and slammed on the brakes my bike slid from under me and I landed on the road head first. I had grazes on both knees and a larger deeper one on the right side of my forehead that bled profusely. Mother sponged lots of grit out of the wound but more grit kept appearing as the wound tried to heal. In the end it left quite a mark, which has never completely disappeared.

Trips on the river Thames had been reintroduced and again it was possible to use these as either a means of transport or simply for seeing the river sights. It was possible to join the boats in Twickenham and either go downstream to Kew, Putney, Hammersmith and eventually Westminster; or go upstream to Teddington (where the first lock was), Kingston, Hampton Court, Shepperton (where the film studios were built), Staines and eventually Windsor.

Father being an Elder of the church we went at least once every Sunday, and sometimes twice, to the Church of Scotland which is on Richmond Green beside the little, and later quite well known, Richmond Theatre. We travelled by train and walked from the station to the back of the church where there was a large hall.

The morning services began at 11 a.m. and before we set out from home Mother would put the complete traditional Sunday lunch of a sirloin of beef, potatoes to roast and two vegetables, as well as a pudding of some kind, into the oven all together on a low heat to cook while we were out. She only had to put the Yorkshire pudding in when we got home.

When I was old enough I went to Sunday School which thankfully took place during the sermon. It is said that Mint Imperial sweets were invented in different sizes, for the different lengths of sermon depending on the denomination. The largest was for the C of S and lasted a good thirty minutes. I felt, early on, that most of the Bible was a good story but that things were being read into the stories that perhaps shouldn't have been. I did not dare express this opinion to my parents, especially Father who took Sunday very seriously.

My parents had a lot of friends. Two that I remember particularly both worked in the newspaper business. Uncle Ralph, as I knew him, had almost black hair and thick black-rimmed glasses. He was a sub-editor of the *Daily Mail*. His wife was the first person that I can remember dying from a condition called 'cancer'.

The other 'Uncle' I knew as Uncle Graham and he had been a Conscientious Objector during the war. As with my father being home all the war, this carried a certain stigma. He could not bring himself to contemplate killing anyone and had driven an ambulance in London throughout the war. I thought that his life was probably one of the most dangerous of all outside the actual armed forces.

We as a family were always doing things, and were quite active. I remained a sickly sort of child. I was just about the smallest in the class and continued to have attacks of infectious diseases or ear problems. I had to have an injection of the newly available penicillin twice a day. I was very thin and my bottom would not take all of them so some had to go into my thigh muscle. The needle was long, and my thigh skinny, with the result that on at least one occasion it struck the bone and bent a needle at an angle of about 30 degrees. I know by this that this is the age I determined to become a doctor.

Father continued in his quest to find a hobby or pastime for me. Rowing was still one of them and of course it was close enough to go and watch the University boat race each April at Putney or Barnes. I expressed no interest in the Cub or Scout movement then, nor at any time. I did take an interest in cricket, and in particular scoring which I began to do for the school. There was a Test match at the Oval and I took myself up one day and practised scoring that match. I was lucky in that that was the match where Bradman was playing magnificently.

The Olympic Games, the first since the end of the war, were held in London in 1948. There was a school outing for a day and I managed to get a few autographs but not of anyone famous, as I recall, as our visit was early on in the Games.

We had not had any pets except the hens until we got a cocker spaniel which we christened Scamp. My early memory of him was his wearing a clothes peg to keep his ears up and out of his food when he was eating.

In this post-war period travelling around the country became possible again and we went up to see Mother's brother, Uncle Jim, who lived in Shaw, near Manchester. On all occasions we travelled by train as, of course, we still did not have a car.

The decision to nationalise the railways had been announced in 1947 but for some time the locomotives and the coaches retained the liveries of the four great companies. Eventually the whole lot became uniformly drab and dirty. As with most of the other public sectors that were nationalised the service became appalling, and the staff uninterested in their customers.

Shaw, where Uncle Jim was a General Practitioner, was a depressing place, seemingly always raining, although the surrounding countryside was quite beautiful. I got on well with Joyce, but Barbara was not easy to get on with. Uncle Jim had built a special double garage to house a huge oo-gauge train layout with lines that went outside and ran round the garden in the summer.

Another model railway, but 1-gauge, was at Beaconsfield near home in London. This was a complete model town that it was possible to walk through. The railway was the most fascinating for me although there were other things like rivers, canals, docks and even a small airport. Legoland, when it was eventually built in Denmark, was in the same style but much bigger.

Holiday trips that I recall were to Teignmouth in Devon in the Cornish Riviera Express, and Porthcawl in Wales. The former I recall as a wonderful place to be in the summer and the latter a really dreary place in the rain. The only good memory of Porthcawl I have is of the funfare and the big dipper.

To visit Scotland we travelled by train from Euston or King's Cross. The LMS line from Euston to Glasgow Central was, and still is to this day, a slow and not very exciting trip. The route from King's Cross to Glasgow Queen Street was via Edinburgh. The train was called the 'Queen of Scots', was also a Pullman and still runs today. It is with amazement that I recall these trips as Father would hire a compartment for ourselves. Food and refreshments were served by the attendants in the compartment. I know that his salary at that time was still well under £1,000 a year.

On these trips we visited Uncle Douglas who was now managing a shipbreaking yard on the Gareloch. I remember the sad sight of the battleship *King George V*, several aircraft carriers and many smaller vessels at anchor awaiting the welder's torch. This visit led to my very first published article in the school magazine, *The Mallian*.

The main idea behind Prep Schools such as The Mall, apart from achieving a pass in the common entrance exam at the age of eleven to gain entry to the secondary school of the parents' choice, was to get a very wide education. It is for the legacy of this that I shall be ever grateful to Mr Ellis and his staff. No matter what is said by politicians and teachers this is not achieved by today's education.

My report at the end of each term was almost guaranteed to incur Father's wrath as I was at one stage in late 1948 under threat of being kept back a class in view of my mixed performances. I have still got a collection of old reports from those days and they make embarrassing reading. My marks tended to hover round the bare pass level but it was the comments section by the Headmaster that usually really riled my father.

In the end I did not get to sit the eleven plus as Father was transferred back to Scotland in November 1949 to open a new branch of the bank in Aberdeen, as Manager. This put paid to his original scheme for my secondary education and it was to turn out to be a very different type at the end of the day.

CHAPTER SIX

Aberdeen, 1949–1953

FATHER started his new job in Aberdeen in November 1949, leaving Mother and me yet again on our own. On this occasion it happily turned out to be for only five weeks as we followed on 4 January 1950. The move to Aberdeen was a major upheaval and I looked upon the move with a mixture of excitement and trepidation.

We arrived in Aberdeen in time for me to start school at the beginning of the new school term, although the rest of the class had started together in the previous August. The school terms, in Scotland, start earlier than in England. My insertion into a new school, in a very different country, in the second term of a new intake was a very bad start for me.

We bought a large detached traditional Aberdeen house in Hamilton Place which is just beside the famous Beechgrove Garden studio of the BBC. It was built in the Scottish Baronial style with the local grey granite from which all of the original city (pre-oil) is constructed. Hence it is known as 'The Granite City'. Number 60 was a corner house on a cross roads with similar, but bigger, houses on two of the other corners and the end of a terrace of town houses opposite us on the fourth corner.

There was a moderate sized garden but not nearly as large as ours in Twickenham. The main difference was the lack of a vegetable patch although there was a conservatory off the back study which, as this was where my parents tended to live, and smoke, became known as the 'snug'. The telephone number was 21843.

At the end of the garden was an old coach house with room for two horses and with an upstairs hay-loft. We were told when we moved into the house that this was an unsafe building and would need to be demolished in the forseeable future. When I visited the area in 1998, far from having fallen down, nearly fifty years later it had been recently converted into a 'yuppy' home with lots of glass, additional rooms and a new roof.

The front door and entrance hall were on the left of the house so that there was only one large room, the dining room, on the front right. My bedroom was above the front door and had the turret which had a small window in it allowing me to watch what was going on at the crossroads and along the street to the bowling green. There was a steep

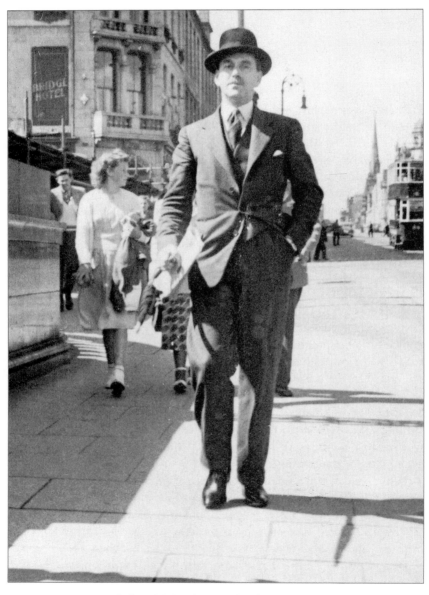

Father. Union Street, Aberdeen, 1950.

staircase to the top floor that had two rooms at the back and one at the front with dormer windows.

The house backed onto another smaller semi-detached version of the same in which lived the Duncan sisters, Sissie and Connie, who seemed to be in their seventies when we moved there but lived for many years without appearing to age any further. They were directly opposite the BBC and along their road was a tram route. There were few buses in Aberdeen in those days but one of the routes crossed the end of Hamilton Place and went past my new school. The bus fare was a halfpenny each way but as it was downhill all the way I tended to walk and save the money to buy sweets which, at this time, were still rationed.

Aberdeen Grammar School was very different from the grammar schools in England that were looked upon by my parents as a last resort. Aberdeen Grammar was the equivalent of a private school but had been caught up in the nationalisation rush and had become a local council school just before I arrived.

It was a very large, all boys, school whose main building was a massive example of Scottish Baronial architecture with a tall clock tower. There was a more modern block, a junior school block, and a new gymnasium. The majority of the boys were day boys but there was a small boarding school about half a mile away.

I had been brought up to consider myself Scottish but of course I returned there speaking like an Englishman and suffered at the hands of the school bullies, and some of the teachers, as a result. My lessons in survival from London helped me cope with this quite well.

I had been doing French in London for some years and was therefore, in my opinion, quite good at it but the teacher was most sarcastic about the way I pronounced the words because of my 'English' accent. This led me to start to become very shy at speaking out in class.

The gym teachers, the Hunter brothers, I considered completely sadistic. They took great delight in taking it out on the least enthusiastic or sports minded in the class. I was still just about the smallest in the class, right up until the age of fourteen, and not really being interested or proficient in any form of sport, suffered badly.

In the summer holidays of 1950 I returned to Holland, this time on my own. I travelled down from Aberdeen by train on either the Flying Scotsman or the Elizabethan. Both these trains started with two or three carriages in Aberdeen to join the main train in Edinburgh.

I again flew KLM but this time I had a label attached to the lapel of my blazer. Although I was thirteen I was still very small for my age and looked younger. Uncle Jo met me at the airport again. They were still living in The Hague but on this occasion I was old enough to get round on the trams on my own. On one occasion I went down to the sea front at Scheveningen and got caught with a full bladder, from too much Coca Cola, in a traffic jam on the way home.

At the beginning of the next school year the powers that be decided

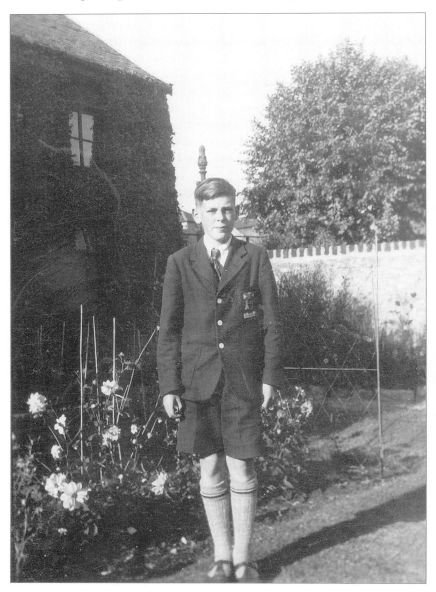

Aberdeen Grammar School uniform.

that they would allow us dissidents to play hockey. I leapt at the chance and, much to my amazement, was good at it and when a first eleven was chosen was included as a halfback. This had enormous implications as there were both home and away matches against other schools, and some of these were girls' schools!

We were very gentlemanly and stuck to the rules. The girls were not at all ladylike and did not stick to the rules. Once our goalkeeper was knocked out. I faired no better in that I was struck across the back of my right hand and three of my metacarpals were broken. So ended my short career in the first eleven. The only bonus for me from all this was that I had to do neither gym nor sports for quite a long time.

My time at The Mall had given me a good grounding in the Three 'Rs' and I was quite good at essay writing. Two of these had a memorable effect on my life. The first was for a competition run by the *Scottish Daily Mail* at the time of the Festival of Britain in 1951. This was a National Current Affairs competition and much to my surprise I won a place in the final. The prize was a four day visit to the Festival itself, in London.

The second essay had an adverse effect on my life. We had been allowed to write an essay on a subject of our own choice. My relationship with the Hunter brothers had reached a level of open hostility and paranoia and I chose to write on the subject of 'Compulsory Games'. In this I let my pen express my personal views both on the subject and on the way it was administered by the Hunter brothers.

I was surprised a few days later to be summoned to the headmaster's, Mr Robertson's, room where I found myself confronting not only him but the Hunters as well. I was given a good dressing down for daring to write this sort of essay and told that this was subversive. I was not to do such a thing again under threat of severe punishment; the strap and the cane were still in common use.

A school in Denmark was twinned with schools in Aberdeen and an exchange visit was arranged in the summer of 1952. Those to be selected to go were from those who could give demonstrations of Scottish Dancing. I was lucky to be chosen among twenty-five from both our school and the other boys' school in Aberdeen, Gordon's College.

We drove to Newcastle in a bus and then crossed the North Sea to Esbjerg in the old steamer *Parkeston* which was used for transporting butter, and bacon, to the United Kingdom and returned empty. On the way out we slept in the hold which was like being in a huge cavern smelling of bacon. From Esbjerg we took the train that has to be split up to be put on the ferry across the Great Belt between Zealand and

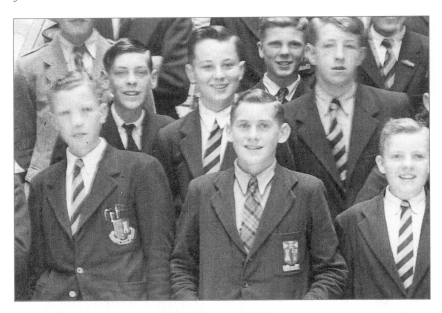

Danish trip, 1951.

Jutland. Now a bridge has been opened in 1998 I do not think it will hold the same excitement.

The family I was staying with lived in the northern outskirts of the city in Charlottenberg. I had a wonderful time there and we did a private exchange later.

We bought our first motor car, a 1937 Austin 10 hp Cambridge with the registration DOA 950. She was known as *Dora*. She was a very sturdy car, which was just as well considering what she was going to have to put up with over the next few years. Although they were fairly basic as cars and black, as they all were, she had a sunshine roof, but no radio.

Father had not ever sat, nor did he ever sit, a driving test 'and proud of it'. He was an appalling driver. He never knew which gear he was in and would stir his hand round above the gear stick until he made contact with it. Mother, on the other hand, had sat a test and was a good driver. I always preferred it when she was behind the wheel.

Dora enabled us to get out and see the countryside of Deeside, Donside, Peterhead, Fraserburgh, and the north coast round Elgin and Cullen, where my father had been brought up. We went for many picnics at weekends and made special trips to Braemar for the Games, and to see the Royal Family.

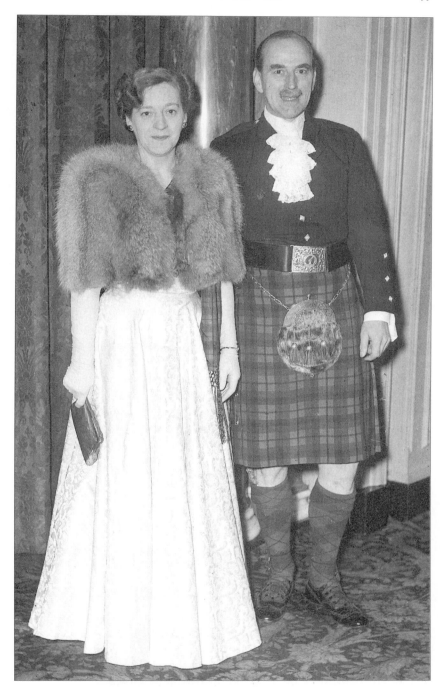

Mother, and Father in kilt, 1952.

We joined Rubislaw church, not fifteen minutes' walk away. The minister was a Mr Lawerence. Father continued as an Elder and I became a Deacon and joined the Bible Class. I thought of it as a normal part of our lives.

Father continued to persevere in trying to find an outside interest for me. In the end it came about more by accident than planning. He and I had gone down to the harbour in Aberdeen, which was always a source of interest, to see the ships coming and going and the large, as it was then, trawler fishing fleet. We noticed a group of boys in a large rowing boat whom I had assumed were Sea Scouts. In fact they were Sea Cadets, which is a completely different organisation and is linked directly to the Navy.

They were in a whaler, which as its name suggests is derived from boats used in whaling, has pointed bow and stern and is rowed by the strange number of five oarsmen. The odd one out is the bow oarsman who also acts as crew for tying up etc and has a shorter oar than the others. It is commanded and steered by a coxswain.

I showed interest in this pastime so Father immediately drove round to their headquarters at the entrance to the harbour and organised for me to look round the following Friday night. I was immediately hooked on this organisation and spent the next ten years associated with it in one rank or another. Father also became keenly interested, joined the parents' association and soon became treasurer.

In the summer we spent a lot of time, often all weekend, learning the skills of rowing the whaler, paddling kayaks the same as the ones used by the famous Cockleshell Heroes, and most exciting of all, sailing. This was a complete new experience for me and I quickly became really interested in this and for the first time in a sport or hobby realised that I had a certain natural flair. I was able to sense the wind and tide flow in some quite inbuilt way.

One of the many spin-offs was the invitation to do collections for charity during the showing of the many 'heroic' naval films that were common in those days. The first one was the 'The Gift Horse' in September 1952 at the Odeon, Aberdeen.

We also learned rifle drill with an old Lee Enfield 303 with the firing-pin removed. I was good at this and soon chosen for the guard of honour. This involved lots of practice and also polishing buckles etc, blancoing webbing belts and gaiters and cleaning the rifle till it shone. To do this we were allowed to take them home on the bus! We got invited to take part in the Coronation Parade in Aberdeen in May 1953.

At the time of the Coronation of Queen Elizabeth II the Sea Cadet

Corps ran a competition, based on drill, to go to the Coronation Review on 15 June 1953 at Spithead. After a lot of stiff competition and hard work I won a place. We were on HMS *Wakeful* (F 159), an old frigate that was in use as a training ship, in line 'E' about two thirds of the way along and the *Britannia* passed close to us. It certainly was a spectacle to remember and unlikely to be repeated, in terms of size, again. The Jubilee Review in 1977 was less than half the size.

The prize possession of the Unit was a motor launch. It was the aim of all of us who had become 'hooked' on boating to be chosen as the full-time crew of this launch.

Once a year the launch would go on a summer 'cruise' that was akin to Scout Camp. This meant going north to the Caledonian Canal, or south to the Firth of Forth and Leith. I was chosen in July 1953 to go on one of the latter, which was to be a week's trip with the object of going from the Forth to the Clyde by way of the Forth–Clyde Canal which was still operational at the time. The first night we stayed in Arbroath and the following morning set off across the open sea directly to the Forth. A fog came down and when we made landfall it was at Seahouses in Northumberland.

The following month Father was promoted and moved again, this time to the Inverness Office to replace his old friend and mentor James Laurie. He had to start almost immediately and went up at the beginning of August.

At the end of August I went to Holland again on my own for a fortnight. This time I flew from Heathrow airport to Schiphol in a British European Airways Viking. As we came across the Dutch coast we flew through a thunderstorm and lightning hit the starboard wing. It spread out over the wing like a golden liquid and I thought that the engine would catch fire as it used high-octane petrol. A slight fire was quickly extinguished, the engine stopped, the propeller feathered and we landed safely. I was somewhat shaken and not greatly impressed with this latest experience of air travel.

Uncle Jo had been promoted to Minister for Welfare for Gelderland, the centre of which is Arnhem. After the war, there had been a lot to do and one of his main tasks was the rehabilitation of the many orphaned and maimed children. He established camps where these children could go and have a holiday much like a junior Butlins.

He took me to one in some pinewoods towards the German border to ensure that all was in order for a visit the following day by their Queen. There was a mixture of excitement, and panic among the staff and the children, some of whom had dreadful injuries. It is an interesting thought that Uncle Jo had been involved in caring for such injured children fifty years before Princess Diana. The visit went off without a hitch although the Queen was seen to shed a tear or two when she saw some of the injuries.

Although I did not actually meet her I have always been in her debt personally. On the day I was to leave Uncle Jo was due to take me back to Schiphol and put me on the plane home. About two hours before we were due to leave their house there was a phone call from the palace to say that the Queen was calling a privy council meeting at 2 p.m. I remember clearly that without a moment's hesitation Uncle Jo pointed out that at that time he would be putting me on a plane.

Asked who it was that was sufficiently important to warrant asking the Queen to change the time of the meeting Uncle Jo explained that I was the son of his colleague Mr Wilson from the war days in London. The caller asked Uncle Jo to hang on and returned a few minutes later to say that in that case the Queen was pleased to delay the meeting until 3 p.m.! The working of the Bank in exile was of some significance to the Queen.

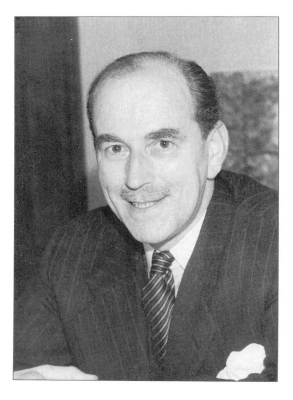

Father, 1953.

The new school year was about to begin and as the Scottish exams were about to be upon me it was decided to put me into the boarding part of the school, better known as 'The Bug-House' on Queens Road, while Mother tried to sell No. 60. In Inverness there was a beautiful Bank house tied to the job.

In anticipation of his improved finances they ordered their first new car, a Morris Oxford. As there was still a steel shortage after the war and lots of other things were in short supply there was a waiting list for them.

Things were not to go to plan, yet again, as Father died suddenly from a massive heart attack at work a month later on 15 September 1953.

It had happened at lunchtime and, as Mother was not at home, I was the first to learn about it by being summoned to Mr Robertson's office in the early afternoon and to be asked if I knew where Mother was. Luckily I knew she was visiting the Sorleys, good friends of my parents who lived a few miles up Deeside, at Banchory. He was a retired General Practitioner and I was ever grateful to him for breaking the news, and to both of them for comforting Mother and getting her back to Aberdeen.

Thus our lives were changed forever. The extent of this change was not to be revealed for some time but I immediately left the boarding house and returned to No. 60 to help Mother.

CHAPTER SEVEN

Picking up the Pieces, 1953–1955

I GOT OVER FATHER'S DEATH quicker than Mother did, or so I thought. Only when I was writing the last chapter did I discover that I had been on the trip to Holland two weeks before Father died. It must have been blotted from my memory and only jogged when I found the map of Arnhem district, annotated with the trips and dates, that Uncle Jo had taken me on.

Mother was inconsolable at her loss and I really believe that she never did recover from it for the rest of her life. She was only thirty-nine when Father died and today she might have been expected to remarry. This subject was never on her agenda, although she was to have several serious admirers.

Father and I had never been particularly close, maybe because of the numerous, and at times prolonged, periods of total separation. During the war years he was always out of the house for one reason or another. He was a very strict man and got riled fairly easily. I was often saved from his serious wrath by Mother's intervention on my behalf. Unlike his father and one of his brothers, I do not think he had any evil in him, just that he seemed very aloof and not easy to talk to.

It had only been in that last year that we had any semblance of adult conversations. I was just learning about his wicked sense of humour and good fun, that Mother was always able to keep as a precious memory. I only heard him use the 'F' word twice. The first time was in London when a taxi he was hailing failed to stop even though it was free. The second time was when a Jehovah's Witness called at No. 60 and managed to get a foot in the door. Father slammed the heavy oak outer door on his foot with great force while inviting the young man to 'f—— off'.

At sixteen I was still quite young and small for my age but was just beginning to notice girls. On one occasion when we were all going down into town in a tram, standing in the centre aisle, I noticed a pretty girl on the pavement and as I followed her with my eyes noticed that Father was doing the same. Nudging Mother I pointed out that Father was 'ogling' the girl. I shall never forget her comment: 'It's when he stops noticing pretty girls that I shall worry about him.'

My very last conversation with Father was rather strange in that it was as if he had a premonition that something was going to happen to him. He walked me back to 'The Bug House', on the Sunday evening just a few days before he died, and talked a lot about how it would one day be my job and responsibility to look after Mother. With his death it had suddenly become a task that I was to take very seriously for the next years.

A post-mortem confirmed that Father had suffered a major coronary artery occlusion almost certainly leading to an immediate cardiac arrest. This news helped Mother in her grief, knowing that he probably had not suffered. He was cremated a few days later in Aberdeen. A large number of friends and banking colleagues attended and this was a great comfort to Mother. After it was all over we had to get down to the serious task of getting on with life and living.

A number of major problems were immediately apparent. Mother was now deprived of an income to support the two of us. I was approaching a critical time in my education in that I was scheduled to sit my university entrance exams in less than two years to pursue my intended career in Medicine. Could we contemplate me continuing on the previously planned educational route, or did we have to change direction completely?

As she was under fifty at the time of his death, Mother would only receive the 10s. (50p) a week widow's pension after the initial 13 weeks at 26s. (£1.30). This was not nearly enough to continue with our plans for my education.

Mr Kirkwood, our family lawyer, advised us that the house was our biggest asset and that we should not consider selling it in the heat of the moment. Mother, however, in the state of shock and grief, found this advice very difficult to follow. She wanted to sell the house and move into something much smaller.

Ann Hastie, an old friend of the family, persuaded Mother that she should use the house to provide an income by taking in what she termed 'Paying Guests'. With some difficulty, Mother accepted the advice and rationalised it as a possible solution by realising that she was accustomed to entertaining people and preparing meals for fairly large numbers. My parents had always kept an open house and even during the war years our home was referred to as 'Liberty Hall'. We did an inventory of all that we might require to run a guest-house and found that there were more than enough changes of linen for all the beds and adequate china and cutlery.

During these discussions there appeared an advertisement in the local paper, the *Press and Journal*, looking for accommodation for a visiting University lecturer and his wife. This couple, Leslie and Leila Macfarlane, did not in fact come and stay but directed a colleague to us. This was the one and only time we ever used an advertisement to get business for the whole of the next eight years.

The first 'Paying Guests' who arrived the following month, October, were Professor and Mrs Harbison-Ocie, and their son Stanley. He was Professor of History at Detroit University and was in Aberdeen for a sabbatical year. Their son came to school with me but there was little in common between us. He was a completely spoiled American child, doted on by his mother to the exclusion of the poor professor.

They had arrived complete with their own car brought over from the States. It was an enormous red Dodge which 'Prof' referred to as 'my lil' old run-about'. We had clung on to our old car *Dora* in the knowledge that she was an asset that we would not be able to replace having luckily been able to cancel the order for the new car in Inverness.

The following summer of 1954, at the end of his sabbatical, they decided to tour Scandinavia and Germany. They very kindly offered to take me with them. I was away for nearly three weeks and I had the grand sum of £42 to pay for my board, lodging and all extras along the way.

During that summer we extended our enterprise and took in our first Dinner, Bed and Breakfast guests who were initially holiday-makers touring Scotland. They came from all over Britain, and from as far away as South Africa and New Zealand. There are hardly any gaps in the visitors' book for that summer and the remarks left by the guests show that they had enjoyed their stay.

The Harbisons were replaced, at the beginning of the following University year, by the Applemans. He was Professor of Bacteriology from the University of South California and his wife was called Lucille. They also had a son called Milo-Don. He was quite a different person from Stanley and eventually also went on to study medicine. They did not stay with us all year as they missed their central heating so much that they found one of the very few houses with it at the time in Aberdeen and moved away from us in the May of 1955.

They did however remain in touch with us throughout their stay and they came back to Aberdeen on a visit eight years later. As an example of how we became close friends with many of our 'PGs' they also came to my wedding in 1963.

My main roles in the business were a combination of gardener, odd job man and chauffeur. I passed my driving test first time, having been taught by Mother as we couldn't afford for me to have lessons. I parked the guests' cars in our rather limited off-road space at night, and un-parked them first thing in the morning. I drove countless makes and sizes of cars over the years and did not damage one of them, as far as I am aware.

As well as helping Mother to run the establishment I had been struggling to keep up with the work at school leading first of all to the 'Lowers' as they are known in Scotland and ultimately to the University entrance exam, or 'Highers'. I did not do too badly in the Lowers and they included French. Aberdeen, unbeknown to a lot of applicants, to this day requires a language at least at Lower level for all Faculties.

The Higher exams themselves were not a success and I ended with only one instead of the three required. This failure had quite serious implications for me. Firstly I was jeopardising my place at Medical School; secondly I was going to have to sit all the exams again, for a reason that I cannot recall and thirdly, and possibly worst of all, I was now over eighteen and subject to call up for National Service. Mr Robertson, the headmaster, on my final report wrote: 'This boy is not up to University standard'. I was duly outraged and vowed to prove him wrong.

At the time of the 'Summer Ball' leaving do at the Grammar School I invited my first 'steady' girlfriend called Moira. Petting was our limit but some of the others, including my best school-friend George, claimed to 'have gone all the way'. In George's case it seemed to have been true as his father, a local GP, was infuriated when he found a pair of scanty ladies' panties on the back seat of his car one Monday morning as he started his rounds, after George had had the car on the Saturday night.

I was called up for National Service but managed to obtain deferment until after the resit results were known in September. At the same time, however, it was made very clear that I would have to go immediately for the two years compulsory Army training if I failed again. I did not fancy the Army and instead opted for a 3-year commission in the Navy. I volunteered for Fleet Air Arm aircrew and went through all the selection stages, passing the medical (they didn't notice the scar of my perforated eardrum), as well as all the flight aptitude tests, and was accepted.

I was so stung by Mr Robertson's rude comment that I worked very hard and determinedly passed the resits. The day I got my results I called at Mr Robertson's house, which was just up the street, to tell him in person that his opinion about me had been wrong. He was gracious enough to admit that in my case he was pleased to have been proved wrong.

I was later to learn that the intake for pilot training that I would have joined lost nearly half the batch in flying accidents mainly due to an design error in the siting of the throttle and flap levers too close together, causing stalling during landing approaches.

It was one thing to have finally gained the entrance qualifications, and be accepted by Aberdeen University to study for the degree of MBChB, but a different matter, and no small problem for us, to find the money to pay the fees. The fee for the course, lasting six years in those days, was £236 5s. payable in five instalments of £47 5s. with only a matriculation fee in the final year. £38 17s. had to be found to enter the four stages of the MBChB exam to be passed over the six years, £28 for the eight weeks compulsory residence during the final two clinical years and money for books and diverse costs throughout the course.

I was very fortunate to have been accepted as a beneficiary of the famous Carnegie Trust that paid my fees.

Mother and I decided, after much deliberation, that we would 'scrape by' as long as I continued to help with running the guest-house and that we would continue to run *Dora* as long as we could afford to. The insurance premium, for both of us to drive her, was £11 12s. for third party, fire and theft.

In the October of 1965 we took in our third academic 'Paying Guest', Dr Kathleen Edwards, a lecturer in Medieval History. She was a sufferer of Still's disease (childhood acute rheumatoid arthritis). She wore calipers on her legs, and had great difficulty in getting about and particularly upstairs. She also had very severe rheumatoid hands and wore splints on the wrists. Her transport was an electrically powered tricycle with tiller steering. It required to have its battery recharged every night as well as being taken to and from the front door every time she needed it.

At the same time as she arrived in the house I started at Medical School.

CHAPTER EIGHT

Medical School, 1955–1961

I N MY CLASS at Aberdeen University Medical School there were only 65 fellow students compared with an average of 150–200 these days; of these only 30 per cent were females compared with today's 60 per cent. There were a number of 'oldies' who had done National Service, and several from overseas. One female, Miss Hazel Cornforth, announced that she had heard that there were people in the class who 'had got in with the minimum qualifications'. I replied that I was one of them.

My personal transport for the next six years was a sturdy semi-racing bicycle. The lectures were spread out across Aberdeen from Marischal College in the Centre, to the new Chemistry building in Old Aberdeen. Apart from our *Dora*, whom I could only afford for special occasions, there were only three other cars in the whole class. Ian Smith had the largest, an Austin 16, Elliot Williamson had a Morris 8 and George Stephens had an Austin 7.

R.V. Jones, famous as one of Churchill's scientific advisers during the war, was Professor of Physics, a prankster and practical joker. To measure the velocity of an object he fired a .22 calibre pistol down the lecture theatre at three spaced revolving cardboard discs. The prime pranksters in the class were Brian and Ken Grassick.

The first prank I recall was when everyone in the class brought an alarm clock to a lecture, set to go off at 3 o'clock, when the lecture was due to finish. The second was at Christmas on a class outing in the 'Gods' at the local Variety Theatre, the Tivoli. There was one particularly dreadful comedian whom we booed loudly. The Manager tried to shut us up but was no match for our numbers and we only agreed a truce when offered our money back.

My only income for spending money for the previous two years had been tips from guests for carrying luggage, moving their cars and the occasional 10*s*. from Mother when she could afford it. I resolved then to earn money for myself during all the available holidays, which in

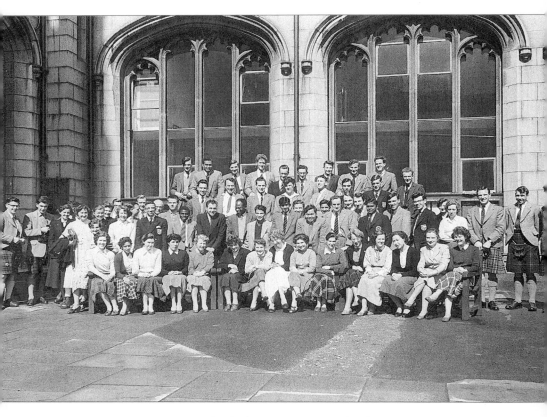

Medical Class, 1955–1961, Aberdeen.

those days were very generous, a month each at Christmas and Easter and three months in the summer.

My social life was strictly limited to a Saturday night out in the University Union bar and cellar Jazz Club. If I had 10s. I felt rich and with £1 I felt very rich. Petrol was 5s. a gallon and beer, bottled McEwan's Export, was 1s. 3d. a bottle. I got seriously into the jazz scene and eventually I became a sort of permanent odd-job man. We had some wonderful evenings over the years and I took up the clarinet myself.

At the Fresher's Evening I had been taken with the Fencing Club's demonstration and decided to take up the Foil. Much to my surprise I was good at it. I began to win matches as I was quick on my feet and my reflexes were pretty good.

At Christmas I worked in the Post Office. I began with the worst task, that is the home delivery, and trudged round some of the housing estates on the outskirts of the city in some appalling weather. After ten days, however, I was put into the registered parcel office in the main post office in Crown Street.

People were sending bottles of alcohol through the post with nothing except a thin wrapping of brown paper and expecting them to arrive in one piece. We often had a row of upturned broken bottles dripping the contents, through the paper, into mugs. All the Scottish banks sent their old bank-notes in small canvas sacks containing £20,000 each on a Friday and, if stolen, would not have been missed till the Monday.

There seemed to be no end of strikes. I got involved with two providing me with an opportunity to drive vehicles not readily available. The first was during a coal strike in the city, when I drove a steam lorry. In the other I drove a tram, but not the large new trams known as the 1938 Aberdeen Streamline.

In the Easter holidays I went to work as delivery driver for a large local grocery firm, Gordon and Smith's, who had been customers and good friends of Father's. I had to deliver a box of groceries to the house of one of the girls I knew from school days. She came to the door, took the box without a further word, and shut the door in my face. I had learned yet another lesson in humanity and politeness.

One of the great events in the students' year was the Charity Week which occurred in the last week of the Easter holidays. A Charities Queen was chosen like a beauty contest and the climax of the whole exercise was the Charity Parade through the City on the Saturday. Dundee University also held their Charity Week at the same time and we would kidnap their Queen for a ransom, and they would do the same with ours. The two Queens were told of the plans in advance so that no one got upset.

A Variety Show was put on at the local theatre, His Majesty's, a full size theatre seating 1,500 people. I was very interested in taking part but as I was inherently still very shy preferred a backstage job. I was asked if I would like to be the Assistant Property Master. Not having an earthly idea what this was or entailed, I simply said 'thank you'.

It was one of the best instant decisions that I have made in my life and for the next five years I lived theatre and 'The Show'. Every day of the holiday was taken up with the writing, production, dressing, staging and rehearsing. The theatre's full-time staff, especially on the technical side, was in charge for the actual performances. I had to scrounge anything and everything that was needed for the production from large bits of furniture to small hand props. I also had to find food and other sustenance for the whole cast, during rehearsals, who were mostly as poor as me. The two local bakers Strathdees and Mackies ran a 'seconds' side of their businesses and we got fruit from traders each day. To move all this food and the properties around I took the front passenger seat, and the rear seat, out of *Dora* to produce a sort of van. I found this entitled me to a petrol allowance from the Show finances.

In that first year show which was called 'Here's to Tomorrow', I met and dated an arts student called Jean Hutcheon. Her father James, who I really liked, was a local General Practitioner.

The first year's study was very boring for me being largely a repeat of the last year at school but meant that the course was six years long. I mainly had to revise and so did not have any trouble with the term exams. The Fencing Club picked me for the team to train for the following year's inter-university matches and as a result I had to put in extra practice sessions. I found that I was not keeping up with my study and so pulled out of fencing so as not to jeopardise my chances of passing the 1st MB first time, which I did.

I finished the year and looked forward to the next one when we started Medical learning in earnest. In the summer vacation I had to earn some money and saw an advertisement for summer staff at Peebles Hydro Hotel, in the Borders, 40 miles south of Edinburgh. I travelled there by train for 8s. 2d. (41p) for a 3rd class return.

I shared a double room with a middle-aged waiter of small stature and balding head. It was plain from the start that he was, as they said in those days, 'queer'. I made it clear immediately that my preference was for the ladies. I thought that he might take offence with this outspokenness but in fact we got on really well.

My first job there was in the Bannockburn bar that was, and still is, the main bar in the hotel. I enjoyed the work there and there were quite good tips which were a vital requirement to make up for the paltry wages we were paid. One of my main failings in education was my inability to do mental arithmetic and the till was badly short.

I was transferred to the dining room where I became 'commis' to the assistant head waiter, a Pole called Nicki. He was a typical gaunt Pole worrying about what was going on back in Poland as he hadn't been able to go back at all after the war, for 'political reasons'.

I got one day off a week and usually was so tired that I just spent it locally walking along the river, or into Peebles town. We were not allowed to fraternise with the guests or their daughters. One daughter took the matter into her own hands and asked me to go for a walk with her on my day off. I did so and we set off up the hill behind the hotel. I was still a virgin and so naive that I did not suspect what was to come until she lay down on the grass. Not wishing to lose out on an interesting lesson I did my best to oblige but when asked why I didn't undo her bra I had to admit I lacked the skill. She immediately stormed off down the hill back to the hotel.

One father handed me a five pound note and asked me to take his daughter down into Peebles. In those days the bars shut at 10 p.m. except if there was a dance with a bar licence. This girl also seemed to be a sex maniac and clutched me close to her bosom, while standing on my feet with her heavy walking boots.

This job gave me experience of life in general, the hotel and catering trade, and human behaviour in particular. The customers were full of complaints, some justified and some simply fabricated. A common one was to complain about being given margarine and not butter 'at this price to stay here'. Of course it was butter all the time so we gave them margarine instead. Another common one was of cold food; as this was rarely if ever the case we would take the plate back into the kitchen, count to 5 or 10 and return it to the table. This was often repeated with underdone, or overdone, steaks and that got the same treatment. No one noticed.

I did learn how so much of the left-over food was recycled. A case of Arbroath smoked haddock lay against the wall outside the kitchen for several days until it was really ripe. The next day it had gone and there was kedgeree on the breakfast menu. The staff were provided with much inferior food and so we learned how to store unused courses from the seven-course *table d'hôte* menu; added to this was the left-over wine and life became a little more tolerable.

The hotel was sometimes asked to do late night dinners for a special occasion and one that is imprinted on my mind was held by some senior Police Officers from Edinburgh. Nicki generously offered to split the tip with me for helping him. At the end of the meal the Chief Constable, who was by now in no fit state to drive back to Edinburgh, asked for the bill (pun). Nicki presented it on a silver plate, a cheque was written, and a silver sixpence (2½p) dropped on to the tray. I sensed Nicki's blood pressure rising; it was nearly 1 a.m. by this time. Nicki dropped the coin on the table and said, 'Thank you, sir, but it looks as if you need this more than we do.'

The very large round metal trays that the hotel issued were heavy fully laden and there was a knack in carrying and balancing them. There were two really spectacular crashes both by girls, exacerbated by their high heels. The first was going into the kitchen with a tray piled high with dirty plates when her feet went from under her and the plates took off upwards followed by a terrific crash of breaking china.

The second occurred when another girl came out with a fully laden tray of a main course and tripped on the edge of the carpet. She fell flat on her face but the dinners continued in a graceful arc across the dining room in a swathe across several tables of diners to distances roughly proportional to their weight. We found peas on the far side of the room under the windows. The poor girl had hysterics and the hotel was faced with quite a large dry cleaning bill.

After five weeks I decided I had had enough. I was working all hours and only able to save about £6 a week. I did not regret the experience as it has held me in good stead on many occasions in my life since. I stayed at the hotel many years later when Nicki was still there.

I spent the rest of the summer helping Mother with the guests and painting much of the outside of the house. As a result I embarked on a career of painter and decorator to many of our friends in Aberdeen and over the next few years this considerably enhanced my income.

We studied Anatomy, Physiology and Biochemistry for the next two years. A good car mechanic cannot possibly mend something if he does not understand how it is made and functions when it is new and in good working order. I cannot understand today's curriculum which does not seem to address this issue.

Anatomy, the structure of the human, is not a subject that changes much in its content but the method by which it is taught can make a lot of difference to its understanding. Together with Embryology, the development of the human form from conception, and Histology, the microscopic appearances of the normal and the abnormal of the organs and other structures, if taught in a manner which links the development stages with the final structure can make the understanding of clinical abnormal presenting signs and symptoms in practice so much simpler.

The Professor of Anatomy, Professor Lockhart, had written his own textbook. The dissection photographs and the accompanying drawings had all been done by members of his own department and were of a quality and style that certainly I appreciated. To extend his vision of teaching us to understand structure and function, he had written a textbook of applied anatomy which linked movement to the muscles and joints that performed the movement.

To give us a sight into the actual shape, position and movements of organs a few of us were X-rayed. They found that my stomach was very long, thin and J shaped in that it went right down into my pelvis before returning to the duodenum. They also spotted a small bubble of air at the lower end of the gullet suggesting a congenital hiatus hernia that was to become a clinical nuisance later in my life.

The Anatomy Department, better known as 'the Drain' was in the basement at the back of the quadrangle of Marischal College, the second largest granite building in the world. No one can forget their first experience on entering a dissecting room with the ever pervasive smell of formaldehyde which is almost impossible to eradicate from clothes and hands.

This was the very first time in our lives that most of the work was done at our own pace and there was no real control over attendance either. It was immediately obvious to me that unless one kept up with the curriculum it would be very easy to drop behind. Not everyone saw it that way and a number of my fellow students spent a lot of time perfecting their snooker, bridge and poker.

The 'demonstrators' are doctors who are planning to go on to a career in Surgery. One of ours was David Milne and our paths were to cross again, once in the 60s and then again in the late 70s.

Another demonstrator was not so popular. His father was an eminent doctor in the City and he seemed to make as much use of this fact as possible. A group of us lifted his car, a Fiat 500, down the long staircase leading to the department, leaving it marooned at the bottom. He was not amused.

Physiology, unlike the unchanging nature of anatomy, seemed to us to be changing by the month. The majority of the teaching was done by Dr Kosterlitz who had a heavily accented German voice. A lot of the experiments related to muscle activity and we were always pouring chemicals on to bits of frogs' legs to watch the effect. Dr Kosterlitz referred to it as 'Tvitch'.

The third subject, Biochemistry, seemed even more in its infancy than physiology and indeed has changed almost beyond recognition since those days. The head of the department was Professor Kermack, and he was blind.

Since Father's death I continued going to church quite often. I had for some time had increasing reservations about religion in general which had been heightened by our work in Embryology etc which did not fit in my mind with the church's version of the creation of man and I was becoming a Darwinian. On Mother's advice, however, I accepted that I might wish to get married one day in church and thus took Communion on 7 April 1957 just before my twentieth birthday.

The Charity Show this year was called 'College Bounds'. Of the five shows that I was involved in it is the only one for which I have not got the souvenir programme. I know that as Property Master I essentially did what I had done the previous year but with an assistant to help me with the running about.

The end-of-year exams at the end of the summer term I passed with my usual sort of average mark, i.e. just over 50 per cent in all subjects except to my great surprise I was getting between 60 and over 70 per cent for all parts of the Anatomy exam. Delighted with this and the thought of a carefree summer ahead, I looked for a job.

Dr Edwards had stayed with us for two full University years and Mother was finding looking after her really quite exhausting. As well as her physical disabilities she was a very demanding person. We decided that we could just not cope with her for another year and had a very embarrassing time telling her that she would need to find new accommodation for the October term.

My unofficial Godfather, and *in loco parentis*, was one of our neighbours across the street, Martin Nichols. He was one of the two local neurosurgeons and was an eccentric. He had been captured with the Highland Division at St Valéry and, like so many of the medical staff, had elected to stay behind with the wounded rather than even try to escape. The Germans must have wished on many occasions that they had not got him as he caused them endless trouble. He taught himself many things while in captivity including Russian, and took part in a number of Brain of Britain contests, reaching the final on at least one occasion.

He was very forgetful about everyday matters. He did a clinic once a month in Inverness. He would drive up and get back late at night. Unable to see his car outside the house the next morning he would report it stolen to the Police. Knowing him of old, they would ask him where he had been the day before and would then check that his car was still safely parked outside Raigmore Hospital, Inverness. He had returned to Aberdeen by train.

One of the other peripheral clinics he did once a month was at Stracathro Hospital, 35 miles south of Aberdeen. He suggested that I apply there to work as a ward orderly where they always needed a few extra in the summer to cover holidays. It was quite hard work involving long hours with an early start on the wards. Coffee had to be made mid morning in the ward kitchen, as well as the afternoon tea. I was posted to the little private patient villa that was well away from the rest of the wards. Here the patients were in single rooms and everything had to be done on an individual basis with trays, tea pots etc. It had its perks, of course.

The hospital, being isolated, had a very active social scene both within the grounds and also in the pubs of Edzell, a village a few miles away. I did not have any girlfriend at that time although one of the physiotherapists took pity on my acne and gave me a course of ultraviolet lamp treatment.

I was really enjoying this life when I overdid the partying in Edzell one night and drank far too much. Being on duty the next morning at 6 a.m. I took two APCs (Aspirin, Phenacetine and 'Codeine) before going unconscious on my bed.

I woke up being violently sick and it still being dark did not at first realise that I was bringing up fresh blood in quite large amounts. I got to the canteen/kitchen where I vomited some more blood over the floor. I was whisked off to the male medical ward and put into bed with some sedation. My haemoglobin turned out to be 47 per cent, as it was measured in those days, of my estimated total.

I was under the care of an elderly, crusty, consultant physician in his last year of practice who did not believe in blood transfusion in someone of my age. I was put on Ferrous Sulphate tablets with a sloppy 'Gastric 1' diet. This consisted mainly of steamed fish and scrambled eggs.

The sister in charge was a real bitch and took it out on me for being a stupid medical student. This immediately endeared me to the rest of the nursing staff who then did their utmost to make my stay bearable. Bed baths by the senior nurses, two at a time I hasten to add, were quite a giggle but the sister tried to extract revenge for this flippancy by sending a poor first year nurse to give me an enema.

She had been persuaded that I had to hold the enema for a considerable length of time before she was to give me the bedpan. Only when I could hear all the giggling going on on the other sides of the screens did I cotton on and gave her till the count of ten or she would have a very dirty bed to change. She, and I, just made it with seconds to spare.

After three weeks I negotiated that I be transferred to Aberdeen Royal Infirmary. I talked the ambulance crew into going past Hamilton Place on the pretext of needing some clean pyjamas. I went into the house to see Mother and then adamantly refused to come out again back into the ambulance. I made a rapid recovery with Mother spoiling me and fussing over me. My subsequent barium meal was essentially normal. I had the remainder of the summer to convalesce and was able to start the new year in October, except that alcohol was banned for six months.

We had been very lucky finding a replacement for Dr Edwards as we needed the steady income during the university year. Laura was studying at Dunfermline College of Physical Education ('Dumf') that had just relocated to Aberdeen. She was a lovely girl and extremely naive, even more so than me. She and Mother became more like mother and daughter and she stayed with us several years until she got married.

I passed all class exams first time and, to my surprise, found that my marks in anatomy had remained high and I was awarded no fewer than three 2nd Class Certificates of Merit. Little did I realise how such a seemingly tiny success in my rather difficult life was to have so much importance nine years later.

The Show was called 'April Showers' and I was invited to be Assistant Stage Manager. It was a whole new world for me and I was also working closely with the professionals of the theatre staff for the first time. I rated a paragraph in the souvenir programme where it alludes to my time spent with the chorus and Jean Hutcheon's sister Muriel in particular. She was tall, slim, attractive and a very good dancer with an incredible sense of rhythm.

April 1958 was also to be my twenty-first birthday. The show finished on Saturday the 19th and so Mother and I deemed it more sensible to have my celebration the following weekend. I had a large party at Raimoir Hotel just beside Banchory. There were twenty-six guests, all paid for by us.

I have a low tolerance of whingers and scroungers today who expect everything to be provided for them for no effort in return. Our boarding house, although continually hard work, did provide us with sufficient funds to have a reasonable life and Mother never missed her coffee followed by a drink every Saturday morning in the Caledonian, which used to be THE hotel in Aberdeen before the oil boom.

The third term of the 3rd year saw the start of a completely new list of subjects. They were the para-clinical laboratory subjects of Bacteriology, Pathology and Materia Medica (Pharmacology). This was doubly exciting as some of the lectures were held in the New Medical School which had recently been built on the same site as Aberdeen Royal Infirmary, known locally as Forresterhill. It had been a large greenfield site, just within the ring road, which had been designated as the site for all Aberdeen acute medicine but only the first phase, in traditional granite, had been completed before the Second World War broke out.

In the first half of the holidays I did some more decorating both of our own house and a couple of rooms for friends. For £4 I had booked a flight from Southend to Amsterdam through the Student Travel Club. I travelled south by bus to save money. I have rarely had such a sore bottom, or such bad cramp in the legs. I resolved to save harder and travel by rail thereafter.

Uncle Jo took me round a great deal in his car and I had a wonderful week. I returned home at the end of the first week in September and helped Mother get ready for another year. I excitedly spent some of my money buying Medical and Surgical textbooks (very second-hand of course) for the real Medical School training beginning on 1 October 1958.

There were two further terms of Pharmacology, Pathology and Bacteriology which form the first part of the 3rd MB exam at the end of the fourth year. There was also great excitement and anticipation at entering the wards in our new and pristine white coats and carrying unused stethoscopes, tendon hammers and opthalmoscopes.

The mornings of the first term were spent doing Surgery. The Professor of Surgery was Willie Wilson who was a most gentlemanly person who was about to retire. Two of his Senior Lecturers were not such pleasant chaps, Hugh Dudley and Norman Matheson. In the years since they taught us they both gained a noteriety of their own.

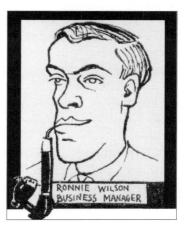

Caricature, 1959.

The majority of Consultants and their junior staff who taught us were pleasant and enthusiastic. Among the senior ones were Bill Michie, Norman Logie and Sydney Davidson and among the younger ones were David Blair, James Kyle, George Mavor (Vascular) and Peter Jones (Paediatrics).

Every morning involved patient clerking in the unit to which we were assigned. The routine of history taking and then the clinical examination was drummed into us by all who taught us so that in a very short time it became second nature to us to do all of it in the same way for all patients. In this way we were unlikely to miss anything of significance. There were no such things as abbreviations.

In the second term Surgery was replaced by Medicine. Professor Fullerton, a quiet, gentle but austere man, was in charge. He was a delightful teacher but we saw too little of him. Our scourge was Dr Tom Morgan who had a vicious temper and would make mock of the person who got answers to his questions wrong. I was never a very forward member of the class and he seriously undermined any attempt on my part to be more outspoken. It was sad then to learn that his mood swings had been due to a slow growing malignant brain tumour to which he eventually succumbed.

The afternoons were split between Pathology and Materia Medica. My most vivid memory of the latter is the demonstration of the efficacy of local anaesthetic. I 'volunteered' to have some injected into my forearm. The lecturer asked if I had felt anything, to which I could truthfully reply 'no'. 'You can look now,' he said and I did; to find that he had pushed a 6-inch nail through the lateral skin fold of my forearm. I promptly fainted! When I came to, on the floor, the nail had been removed and a bandage applied. I have been slow to volunteer since.

The Students' Show that spring was called 'Alma Mania' and I became the Business Manager. It was a demanding job and took up a vast amount of my time. Muriel was by now my steady girlfriend, and everyone in the cast of the Show was aware of our relationship. She spent breaks in the rehearsals knitting me a large red sweater. In this show she danced the solo part in 'Slaughter on Tenth Avenue'.

In the third term of that year we returned to Surgery and the hard graft up to the Professional Exams in Pathology, Bacteriology and Materia Medica. I had to burn the midnight oil in a way that I had not had to in the past but luckily it paid off and I passed the first part of the 3rd MB at the end of the summer term by a margin that can only be described as thin.

I had arranged an elective clinical attachment in Orthopaedics in Copenhagen. In order to fund this I had had to do a lot more decorating for friends of ours. I left from Newcastle to Esbjerg on the *Winston Churchill* on 15 August. I had originally been booked into a students' hostel but after a couple of days I found a flat in 'The Triangle' so long as I was prepared to share with another student from the UK.

My attachment was arranged directly with Professor Bertelsen. The Orthopaedic Hospital in the northern outskirts of the city has 300 beds. I was made very welcome there and attached to one of the two teams that did alternate days emergency and elective work. The day started early and finished, on the non-emergency days, at 2 p.m. Two specialities of the hospital were laminectomy and spinal fusions for children who had had polio.

It was an eye-opener to me to see the 'permissive' way of life in that city. The local students and nurses took me out to all their haunts in the pubs, the clubs and the Tivoli Gardens. Having had no sexual experience up to this time I was amazed at the open display of condoms on the part of the girls especially.

Muriel came to see, and stay with, her old Nanny, Karen. After Muriel had been there a week or so her Mum and Dad came over as well. We showed them the sights, I had a relaxing week and then we all travelled back together. Dr James excelled himself by getting on the wrong half of the train at the end of the Great Belt ferry passage but he was at least on the train.

While I was away Scamp, our cocker spaniel, had died. This loss had left Mother even more lonely, with me away, and so we immediately replaced him with a liver and white springer spaniel whom we named Roger.

The Sea Cadets were very short of Officers and in view of my experience I applied and was accepted on to the books of the Royal Navy as Temporary Acting Sub-Lieutenant Wilson SCC. I received a handsome cheque with which to purchase my uniform which I did from the Merchant Navy tailor in Aberdeen. He made me the very best No. 5 reefer suit in doeskin that was to last me, and my son after me, for over thirty years.

The fifth year began in October. The first of the new subjects was Mental Health, taught by Professor Miller, who did his best to make it interesting, and Dr Sinclair Gieben, who seemed an eminently sensible chap but who committed suicide.

Public Health, or 'drain sniffing' as we called it, was entertainingly taught by Professor Blackett and Dr Richardson. Midwifery, Radiology and Venereal Diseases were the other three subjects included in that term.

The University Rowing Club on the banks of the river Dee had been overwhelmed by new students wishing to join and had no one to teach them. I offered to train a crew but not having a clue as to how to go about this I felt a little foolish when I was allocated four lads and a boat. We spent hours getting the balance right and at the end of the day it all clicked and I had the feeling that between us the five of us might make something of this given enough time.

After Christmas back at University we added Dermatology, Child Health and Infectious Diseases, Ear, Nose and Throat and Opthalmology. The class was divided into three groups for these clinics and the three terms of that year were spent rotating between the three groups of subjects.

The Charity Show in the spring was called 'Folies Berserques' and I, together with my friend John Skene (a year behind me) was Co-Administrator. This is the highest that a student could get in the running of the show. Above that the professionals from the theatre took over. Muriel was not in the show as it was her final year.

At the end of the summer term was an exam in Forensic Medicine and Public Health. These were, to me, two insignificant subjects and I had fallen into the trap of not keeping up with my revision. This together with the over commitment to the show meant that even my burning of the midnight oil did not save me from ignominy and, predictably, I failed miserably.

I was devastated and extremely annoyed with myself but I suppose it was better to be taught a sharp lesson this year rather than the next and final, so I gritted my teeth for the resit in September. Muriel had passed her finals and graduated MA. At this stage she was not sure if she wanted to go to Teacher Training College like her sister Jean.

I had arranged to spend the summer at Stracathro doing a surgical elective. I was a student, not an employee this time, and was accommodated in the 'Mansion House' which was (and still is) a large Georgian house on whose estate the hospital had been built.

Mr Neil Hendry, an Orthopaedic surgeon, like Martin Nichols, did a clinic once a month at Stracathro. His hobby was Alfa Romeos and he proudly used to keep a note on how fast he could get from his home on Queens Road to the hospital. Even in those days it was alarming and I was quite glad not to have been a passenger.

On one occasion Martin Nichols failed to arrive and they immediately asked me where he might be. I phoned his wife Barbara, at home, to discover that he had left on time. Someone had seen his car at Laurencekirk, about five miles north of the hospital, but he was not in it. I set forth in *Dora* and found him at a set of roadworks driving a coal-fired steam road roller.

There was a busy casualty department and the only one for miles around. We used to get horrific multiple traumas. If the patient survived the first few hours, I observed, they usually did well in the end. Years later the term 'the Golden Hour' was coined.

I remember giving my first anaesthetic, and reducing my first Colles fracture on the same patient, at the same time. It was nitrous oxide inhalation and when the patient had gone limp the surgeon suggested I might like to come round and manipulate the wrist. This I duly did, held it till the plaster was applied, and then returned to wake the patient up again.

I remember seeing my first cardiac arrest. A young man's heart stopped suddenly at the end of the operation. Intensive care units were not common and we simply left the patient on his ventilator, in the operating theatre. He stayed there for two days only to recover completely, and suddenly, on the third. He could not believe that he had been unconscious for so long and we had show him the newspaper with the date.

It was a lesson that I have never forgotten; if you don't attempt to resuscitate someone you will never get survivors. I used the same philosophy in my treatment of cancer patients in the future.

I was committed to doing a stint with the SCC supervising a camp in Winchester. In those days Officers, even Temporary Acting Sub-Lieutenants SCC, travelled First Class in Uniform. This was fine until I got repeated asked, especially at King's Cross, for train and platform information. Wardroom life was quite new to me and I got to like getting my first cup of tea brought to me in bed by a steward and enjoyed the routine of dressing for dinner. I certainly decided that this was a way of life that I could go for.

I felt much more confident of the outcome of the resit exams as I felt that I knew what the questions were about and could write about them all. Unfortunately final year started a month early, at the beginning of September, before the results would be available and the thought of starting the year and then having to repeat the 5th year did not fill me with joy.

The first term started with placements with District Nurse home visits and visits to the ante-natal and gynaecological clinics. It was a great relief when during this time I learned that I had passed the resits and that I was going to be able to continue with the rest of the class into the final year proper.

I had to seek, and luckily was granted, a week's leave of absence from the wards as the Navy had found a slot for me to do the Reserve Officers' Qualifying Course on HMS *Sheffield*, the Reserve Fleet HQ Ship, in Portsmouth.

One task on the course was to sail a cutter upwind to a large buoy and deposit one of the officer trainees on it, go round again and pick him up. I managed the manoeuvre without too much difficulty but when it was my turn I spent a long, cold and wet time on the buoy, until I was retrieved.

During our course the Wardroom held the Reserve Fleet's Trafalgar Night Dinner. A notice went up offering two places to the SCC course. After several days there had been no takers and I could not persuade any of the others to join me. I felt there was no point in wasting a valuable learning opportunity when we were on the course anyway and approached the course officer saying I was the only one willing to go. He agreed to sit beside me.

I was totally unprepared for the seniority of the guests, the size of the gathering, the size of the meal and the amount of alcohol to be consumed. I was sat at the end of a long table at right angles to the top table almost opposite the Admiral Commanding Reserves in its centre. My mess kit consisted of my No. 5 reefers and a black bow tie.

There is no smoking until after the meal and the Loyal Toast has been made. This, in the Navy, is taken sitting down because one of the Georges banged his head on a low beam.

The first toast was to Nelson, Trafalgar and the Reserve Fleet by the president of the Wardroom; replied to by the Admiral Commanding Reserves. I was really into the swing of things and feeling this was the life for me.

The next speech was to the guests, in which I, the lone SCC Officer, got a mention. Then the final speech was a reply to this 'by the most junior officer present'. 'I wonder what poor sod that is,' I thought, an instant before the course officer poked me to point out that that was I! By this time the assembled diners were beating the tables and shouting, 'Up, up, up.' There being no escape I rose unsteadily to my feet assisted by the course officer's strong arm but the diners continued to shout 'up', so I climbed onto my chair to thunderous applause and cheering; followed by total silence.

I cannot remember exactly what I said but I spoke in the direction of the Admiral and said I was sure I was speaking for all the other guests in thanking the hosts for the invitation and how much I had enjoyed this, my first Dining Night. I collapsed down onto my chair again, red as a beetroot and sweating profusely, to rapturous cheering and applause and claps on the back from nearby officers.

I had just regained my composure after my ordeal when a voice said in my ear that the Admiral wished to speak to me. My legs returned to jelly. He was a charming man wearing a frock coat, the first I had ever seen, and he congratulated me on my handling of the situation, admired my doeskin uniform, bought me a beer and wished me luck with the rest of the course and my career.

I passed the course and could now be a proper Sub-Lieutenant SCC although I began to prefer to think of myself as being in the RNVR, with the wavy stripes.

Muriel had decided to go to Edinburgh to do a secretarial course and so I did not see so much of her. I think at this stage both Mother and her family took it for granted that we would become engaged but the relationship was going through a bad patch and part of the reason for her wishing to go away from home was 'to get some space'.

After all these years of hard work Mother's health was beginning to suffer and I realised that as soon as I had qualified we would have to take a decision about the future of the house which was going to be far too big for her when I left; and she certainly ought not to carry on the business beyond my final year. She had suffered from myxoedema for years and could never sleep properly without a sleeping tablet, of which

I began to strongly disapprove. She continued to smoke at least twenty a day and usually nearer thirty. By now I knew that this was not good for her and I also noticed that she had begun to get some intermittant claudication if she tried to walk any distance.

This latter she treated with liberal doses of Grant's Standfast whisky and a little water. She could consume several doubles of these with no noticeable effect but it helped her legs. One gin and tonic, however, and she became very morose; one glass of sherry and she became very giggly; two glasses and she was uncontrollable.

It was during this term that I was to lose my virginity. A 6th year girl from St Margaret's Girl's School, who came from Montrose and who had up until then lived in the boarding house of the school, had told her parents that she did not want to be there for her 6th year. Mother had met her and her parents, and agreed to take her in for the year.

This newly acquired nubile boarder was undoubtedly a distraction and started making passes at me especially if Mother was out and we were alone in the house in the evening. On one such occasion this led to the first kiss and she evidently expected more. One thing led to another, and it became apparent that she wished me to go to bed with her. She was partly amused and partly aghast when I explained to her that I was a virgin and was not entirely sure what to do, even though anatomically and physiologically, I knew the theory well. The next time Mother went out to see her friends in the evening she told me she would show me what to do and we repaired to her bed.

I can't say it was earth-shattering, especially as just as I was beginning to enjoy the rhythm, she had a climax and immediately demanded that I withdrew 'before coming'. Having thus experienced *coitus interruptus* in my first sexual adventure, I have never viewed it as a form of contraception to be recommended.

Mother came home early one night while I was still in her bed and was obviously extremely shocked that her paragon of virtue should have fallen so. The girl was told to leave at the end of the week. I was in severe disgrace for some considerable time.

After Christmas, the first that I hadn't worked for the Post Office, our section of the class returned to Surgery and Anaethetics. I enjoyed Surgery but was not really interested in a long term career in that subject as it appeared to me that the trainees had to work extremely hard, had long hours on call, and too much studying to do.

In early March I went to the Medical Ball, for the very first time. Muriel came up from Edinburgh for the weekend. It is only when I look at photographs of those days that I realise how dreadfully thin I was for my height and that I had very sticky out ears. My nicknames ranged from 'beanpole' to 'lamp-post'. It was the days of the Goon Show and I was also known as the 'thule' man. Mainly I was known simply as 'RG'.

The boat crew were performing so well that the club had decided to enter us for the Scottish Universities Open Championship that summer which would involve a lot of travelling round Scotland and the north of England as far south as Durham.

During the spring vacation I had agreed to go to a SCC camp at Faslane, near Helensburgh, which was (and still is) a submarine base,

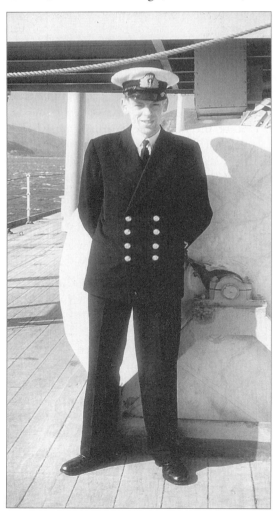

Sub-Lieutenant SCC
HMS *Adamant*, 1960.

for two weeks. The depot ship for the submarine flotilla was HMS *Adamant* that went to sea once a year or so, to be the target for one of the submarine commanders' qualifying courses. This is the course that has been made famous by the TV series 'The Perishers'.

I got involved in bridge watch-keeping. It was an open bridge which was unbelievably cold and windy. As the target for the submarine we were not only zig-zagging but interspersing this with a fine weave on each leg of the zig or zag. In the middle of the night a voice boomed out behind me, 'You were two seconds late with that, Subbie.' Later that night the ship was struck by a dummy torpedo between the rudder and the hull, jamming it. Luckily we had enough sea room to allow us to turn round and round in circles until the torpedo freed.

Back in Aberdeen it was Charities Week but I was not involved this year as I had had my lesson the previous year. Muriel and I went to the Charities Ball at King's College at a cost of two guineas each.

The final term was to be hectic. Our group was now doing clinical Paediatrics together with Obstetrics and Gynaecology. During this latter we had to live, for eight weeks, in the residence just beside the maternity hospital, which was at the foot of the hill from Forresterhill. We had to perform twelve deliveries ourselves and be signed up for them.

The first delivery I ever witnessed was of great embarrassment as the girl was a nurse who I knew, and she wasn't married. She saw me and said, 'Oh Ronnie, how nice of you to come.' Needless to say, everyone in the delivery room assumed that I was the father. The first baby I delivered myself I nearly dropped taking it to the sink to wash it, as it was so slippery and it was a little like trying to remember how to catch a rugby ball. I can't imagine what would have happened if I had actually dropped it.

The Nurses' Home was the target for pranks by those in residence. It was the real old type of nurses' home where the door was locked at some silly early hour and girlfriends were pushed through the windows of the ground-floor toilets.

We introduced a goat through the front door up to the top floor and left it there. It refused to come down again and we had to go in again and collect it. This caused an outcry when males appeared rushing around in the home in the middle of the night. Matron was not amused.

The various boat races meant that we had to travel around with the boats strapped to the top of an adapted coach to the cities that were hosting the races. It was usual to collect souvenirs from the city visited and prime prizes were street names. I was on the top of a pyramid wielding a screwdriver removing a 'Sauchiehall Street' sign in the middle of Glasgow when a policeman came round the corner. He simply invited us to replace the screws as we had found them and to go home. I doubt if that would happen today.

We qualified for the final of the coxed fours that was to be held on the Clyde at the end of the term. We would earn a University Blue if we won so we went into even more serious training.

In Paediatrics a dear child gave me chickenpox which then became evident three weeks before the finals. My face and trunk became covered with a dreadfully itchy rash and Mother covered me with calamine lotion. I made my mind up that I was going to the finals and that was that. Anyone liable still to catch it would have to take their chance.

Much worse was that the final written exams were all day on a Friday and the Saturday morning. That Saturday was the date of the boat race finals in Glasgow. After two years training I wasn't even going to be there and the crew won! Given my lack of sporting prowess in my life I have never really forgiven the University authorities for robbing me of my one claim to sporting fame.

The following week we had the vivas in all the clinical subjects. At the end of the last afternoon we had to queue up at Marischal College to see if our name was on the pass list that was pinned up on a notice board.

Being a 'W' I could start at the bottom and know that if I had passed it would be near the end. It was a great relief, therefore, to find it very quickly third from the end where it should have been. Knowing how much this would mean to Mother I was one of the first to use the phone and tell her the good news. She had almost forgiven me for my indiscretion and I think this put us back on to our old relationship once again.

The Graduation ceremony was the only time I have ever worn a gown. The whole gathering had to sit through every capping and after a while it got a bit boring. I was pleased for Mother as she at last could feel that all her hard work had not been in vain.

There was only a month from then until I started my first house job and I had to discuss with Mother what she was to do now that I had qualified and she no longer had to go on working; nor would she need such a large house. Not surprisingly she didn't really want to move and we came up with a compromise solution which was to turn the house into two flats. Mother would keep the bottom one and sell the top one.

For my 'paid holiday' I had arranged to go for two weeks to the Royal Naval Air Station, HMS *Fulmar* at Lossiemouth to supervise the SCC camp. I was lucky in being able to make friends with the aircrew with whom we shared the wardroom.

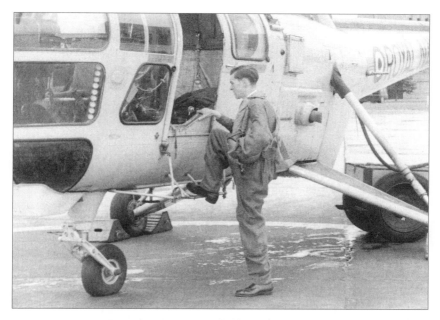

RNAS Lossiemouth, 1961.

Lossiemouth had a flight of S51 'Dragonfly' helicopters and I arranged to go for a flight. The pilot took us up the Spey valley to 'visit' the whisky distilleries. The other passenger was a Naval photographer who was taking aerial pictures for the distillery companies. We stopped at one to be shown round and all but the pilot had free samples. No doubt such things would be frowned on now.

I was also offered a flight in a Hunter T22 Naval Jet Trainer. I had to go through the ejection seat training and show that I could release myself from the seat once ejected and was shot up the ejection escape static tower. I still find it difficult to describe the flight. We headed out across the North Sea towards Norway and then the pilot told me I had control and I thought I was doing wonderfully well but we were climbing almost vertically.

I had just one week on my return to get myself organised to move into the Doctors' Residence at Forresterhill to begin my House Year.

CHAPTER NINE

House Year, 1961–1962

T HE TRANSITION from being a student to a working doctor, and the speed with which it happened, was something of a shock to my system. I shared my Surgical Orthopaedic job with Ed Barron. We were on call alternate nights, the type of regime that I was to experience throughout the remainder of my training. It was something one got used to and I can't say that I ever felt as exhausted or dangerous to the patients as the modern junior doctors claim.

The residence for the housemen (women) was a block near the centre of the hospital. We did not see our room all that much as we were very busy. We found that the food was awful particularly in comparison with that given to the patients. We complained to the Medical Director, Dr Michie, who told us that it was much easier to replace junior doctors than it was to replace a chef and that we could like or lump it ... Maybe he was the prototype of today's managers?

There were 80 beds between the male and female wards and at any one time I would be responsible for 40 of them. The day started early to check the well-being of the patients and to take any blood tests that were needed and this was done by 8.30 a.m. The rest of the morning would consist of ward rounds or attending the operating theatre, as in those days the houseman was expected to be there as the second assistant.

The Sister on the male ward was an archetypal dragon who used to 'eat housemen for breakfast'. She was an obsessive woman and all the loose items of equipment, down to the last pencil, had 'Ward 7' written on them in indelible ink. It was rumoured that she was having an affair with one of the Consultants and I think we would have been able to confirm this, if only from the body language on ward rounds.

Getting all the relevant X-Ray packages out of the X-Ray department in time for the weekly ward round proved well-nigh impossible, although most departments lived with the myth that they could provide the films on demand. Ed Barron and I devised a system where we had a tin trunk under the desk in our office. In this we gathered the X-Rays, in their packets, for the next ward round. The X-Ray department retaliated by sending their secretaries down to take them back. This we stopped by having a large padlock and only two keys.

Ward rounds were the only days that we were given coffee by the ward sisters. We were definitely viewed by them as the riff-raff. It was different once the night staff had come on as in those days a third year nurse would be in charge, with a night sister overseeing a block of wards. A 10 o'clock visit to the ward was invaluable as the nurses had found out if there were any problems, they could be sorted, night sedation written up and drip regimes checked. This would usually result in a cup of coffee being produced by the junior nurse. I am sure this evening routine saved many phone calls during the night except for the unexpected event and practised this throughout my training.

There was mayhem on the male ward one night when it was discovered that a Swedish seaman with a fractured femur strung up in a Thomas's splint and traction, had managed to manoeuvre himself round and was having intercourse with his girlfriend behind the drawn screens. We were full of admiration for his determination but alas, the hospital complained to the Swedish Consul.

On the days that we were expected to be in the theatre it usually entailed holding a retractor for hours on end and being shouted at if you let it slip at all. One day Mr Rennie did something that possibly changed my life. The last case on this particular list was the removal of a screw from an ankle fracture. He handed me the scalpel, without a word. I hesitated for a mere second and took it from him. He told me exactly what to do and I was amazed that once I had begun all my nervousness disappeared.

He told me later that he did that with all his housemen and if they did not accept the scalpel he did not offer it again. In my case he let me do more and more, under his own supervision, and his colleague Mr Adams began to do the same. It culminated just before I finished the six months by being allowed to pin the third of three fractured necks of femur on the list. I got the guide-wire in the right place on the second attempt and took only a little longer for the case than the Registrar, who had done the second one.

I perpetrated a major boo-boo in that job and had the outcome been any different, Mr Rennie's view of me might have changed significantly. A young woman of about nineteen had non-union of fractures of her right forearm bones. It had been decided that they would have to be fixed with plates and screws. I took her blood pressure, listened to her chest and pronounced her fit for anaesthetic. At the beginning of my notes I had written, 'A rather obese young woman for her age.'

Mr Rennie was in the anaesthetic room with the patient when there was a bellow of 'Wilson' and I realised that something was wrong and I'd better go and face the music. I didn't expect to find the girl had gone into labour on induction of the anaesthetic. Luckily for all concerned, the contractions stopped after she had been woken up again and put back to bed. On interrogation she admitted that she had told no one, least of all her mother with whom she lived, that she was nearly nine months pregnant. We transferred her to the maternity hospital where she delivered a healthy boy the following week with no problems.

We were paid the handsome sum of £650 per annum. It had become clear that I would have to have a car of my own particularly before I went off to Stracathro for my second job, if I was to leave Mother with *Dora* who by now was really beginning to be on her last legs and would not be up to repeated long trips.

I had found a 3 litre Red Label Bentley whose owner only wanted £350. I would have had to borrow most of this and they wanted Mother as guarantor of any loan. She refused! At the end of the day I realised that she was quite right but at the time I was miffed especially as one of my non-medical friends had just bought a 1926 Rolls Royce ex-taxi for £250.

The bank did agree to lend me £150 without a guarantor. At the end of August I heard, through Mr Neil Hendry, of a Mk7 Jaguar with low mileage and only one owner, a farmer who would sell it to me for that amount. It was in pristine condition except for the driver's carpet which was in muddy tatters. It would do 22 miles to the gallon if the two carburettors were clean, in tune and the mixture was set right. Otherwise it was liable to do only 16. I spent a lot of time tuning the engine to perfection on alternate weekends using my stethoscope applied to the air intakes.

One Saturday morning, while I was doing this outside the residence, Mr Rennie came past in his fairly new Mk2 2.4 Jaguar. He stopped and admired my car and then said he was having a lot of problems with the engine and that the garage had had several goes at getting it right but without success. I offered to try to make it better and he left it with me for the rest of the day. I stripped the carburettors down, cleaned everything, checked the timing and put it all together again and then tuned it. It sounded like a different car. Mr Rennie was delighted and went round telling everyone that I was his mechanic, as well as his houseman.

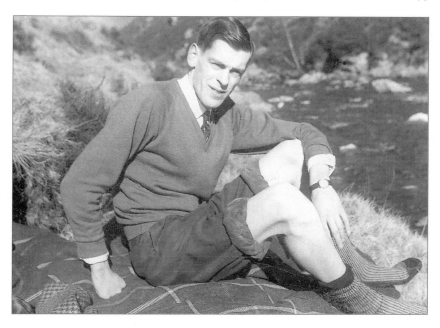

Dr Wilson up Glen Esk, 1962

We had got planning permission to split No. 60 during the autumn and this was followed by estimates for the building work. We were eligible for a grant, or grants, for the alterations and applied for these but this was to delay us until into the New Year. We decided that it was probably better to do the building work in the spring, once the weather had improved.

Muriel had by now moved to London and was working for Unilever as a personal secretary. Our relationship had cooled considerably and I started to seek fresh female company. One of the third year nurses at the time was a flaming natural redhead called Elizabeth. Ours was a good relationship but didn't last very long as when she qualified she went to work in Inverness. Those who know of my liking of real redheads, as opposed to those from a bottle, will now recognise the reason for this.

I drove down to Stracathro on 31 January ready to start the next day. The pace of life in the Medical job was so much less than in the Surgical one. This together with the smallness and friendliness of the actual hospital made it a much more enjoyable six months.

I was on my way back from Arbroath about 1 a.m. one night when I saw a stag in the distance. I was travelling very fast in the Mk7 (i.e. over 100 mph) and immediately started to brake. The stag stopped in the middle of the road so I decided to stay on my side of the road and go in front of him. I was still going uncomfortably fast when he moved forward again blocking the road in front of me. Knowing the outcome of cars hitting stags I wrenched the wheel round and scraped round behind him just keeping on the road in the process. If I had not been sober before meeting him, I certainly was after.

The superb handling qualities of such a large car undoubtedly saved my life in another even narrower squeak. I was returning to Stracathro from seeing Mother on one of my nights off. Near Laurencekirk there are some very sharp bends. It was dark and oncoming vehicles were easily visible at a distance because of their headlights. I saw what I took to be a lorry from the size of the beams, coming towards me and stayed well into my side of the bend, but I then saw a second set of headlights overtaking it on my side of the road.

The only way to avoid a head on collision was to increase the hard left lock and hope that there was a fence, and not a stone wall, at this part of the road. I shot off the road, through a wire fence into a ploughed field as the two lorries passed my rear in parallel. I came to a halt well into the field at right angles to the road. It was soft ground and the car weighed about one and a half tons. I waited until I had stopped trembling, said a quick 'thank you' prayer and another hoping that I could get out again. In fact I simply reversed out very slowly along my tyre tracks, through the fence and back on to the road.

Muriel had written to me and I arranged to go down for a weekend, which meant driving to Edinburgh Airport after work on a Friday and catching the last flight to Heathrow. This was in a British European Airways Vanguard the week after one had crashed on the runway at Heathrow. Muriel and I got on better than we had before she had gone south and I had a good weekend. On the return flight, also in a Vanguard, we went via Glasgow; no one told us why. We flew most of the way on the short hop from there to Edinburgh on three engines as one of them had failed on takeoff.

In April 1962, having got the grants for the house organised, Mother decided to get ahead with the work to divide it. The major work was breaking a new door through the thick granite round the side of the house into the large hallway, turning the bottom of the staircase to face directly down and then dividing the hallway to separate the two entrances.

Mother kept the large ground floor, making a bathroom out of what had been the large pantry and making the 'snug' into her bedroom, with the French door and conservatory off it. She kept the large kitchen, and the outhouse as her wash-house and coal house. The large front room became a lounge/dining room. The only piece of furniture that we regretted having to part with was the grand piano, under which I had slept during the war. We then sold the upper flat, which consisted of the top two storeys, and paid our part of the grant back to the council from the proceeds.

In May I formally applied to the Admiralty, as it was properly called in those days, to do a Short Service Commission and was summoned to Queen Anne's Mansions, St James Park for an interview. I was duly accepted in June and received all my necessary joining instructions and uniform allowance in July. I had to tender my resignation as (still) Temporary Sub-Lieutenant SCC RNR, as it had now become and the wavy stripe was lost forever except for SCC officers.

I resolved that, as I owed Mother so much for her struggle on my behalf, I would take her on a holiday to see some of her friends that she had not seen for a long time. This meant a long trip through Northern Europe. We set off in the Jaguar in the last week of July. The first stop was in Boroughbridge in Yorkshire to see the Graggs. In reality it wasn't the first, or even second, stop, as Mother had developed what I later was to discover a lot of ladies suffer from, a small and irritable bladder. She found it almost impossible to go more than 100 miles without stopping. The timing of some of my travel plans had not taken this into consideration.

Our next drive was to Harwich where we caught the ferry to Esbjerg in Denmark. In Copenhagen we stayed with people who had stayed with us in our guest-house and who themselves ran a small hotel in Klampenborg, just north of the city. We arrived quite late and they were in the middle of serving dinner to their own guests. They sat us down in the kitchen with a bottle of whisky for Mother and beer for me. By the time they were finished and we could all sit down for something to eat and a chat, Mother was very merry and thoroughly enjoying herself in a way that I had not seen for years.

The night before we were to leave when we were all very merry again our hosts pointed out that we had arrived a day after we had said we would and were staying a day beyond. They had taken all in their stride and not complained. We caught up with ourselves again in Svenborg in the south of Denmark on our way to Hamburg to see the Mullers. Mother had not been there before, nor seen them since before the war.

Finally we went to Holland to stay with Uncle Jo and Tanta Nellie in Oosterbeck for several days. That was a very moving reunion for them and of course Robbie, their son, was grown up and going to college.

I think she had really enjoyed herself but was tired out. It had become obvious to me being with her so much that the circulation in her legs was getting much worse and she could only walk short distances without a rest. I had decided that before I left for the Navy I would get Mr Mavor to see her. She had no pulses below the groin and her angiogram confirmed she had severe athero-sclerosis. I already knew the implication was that she would have athero-sclerosis elsewhere, including her coronaries.

He advised her to stop smoking and take a little whisky which would help to increase the blood flow. Mother ignored the first piece of advice, as I knew she would, and accepted the second by doubling her tots per day from two to four.

On 2 September 1962 I set off in the Jaguar for Portsmouth to join 'HMS *Victory* for RN Barracks' the following day.

CHAPTER TEN

Royal Navy, 1962–1965

I MUST HAVE HAD some sort of doubt in my mind about committing myself to even five years in the Navy, let alone sixteen years' Regular Commission, as I restricted my contract to only three years.

My first experience of the Navy proper was at the RN Barracks, Portsmouth, which is just next to HMS *Victory* herself. I was joining a group of other doctors, dentists, teachers and chaplains who all, with their professional training, had to learn as much as possible about the Navy in six weeks.

There were lectures on Naval history, etiquette, regulations, dress regulations, security and intelligence; this last being very interesting as we were still at the height of the cold war. There was a serious possibility of us being compromised or blackmailed by Iron Curtain countries as the Russians had seemingly opened a file on all Gazetted Officers.

There was daily physical training, which I continued to loathe and be useless at, together with basic parade ground drill. This was easy for me but one or two of my colleagues really did have a problem with which arm to swing with which leg. Of greatest amusement was sword drill which was not done with ceremonial swords, probably too valuable, but with heavy cutlasses. Several ears, if not heads, were nearly lost in these classes.

Filling the rest of the time we had training in fire-fighting, the use of respirators in confined spaces (as found on ships), swimming skills such as righting overturned life-rafts (another of my least favourite pastimes) and being taught how to escape from a ditched helicopter by means of a mock-up which was lowered into the water upside down. This latter was awful and nearly finished my short service career on the spot.

We spent some time at sea in one of the frigates of the training squadron seeing how the ship and the various departments worked. Quite a lot of time in the afternoons was spent in rowing or sailing the various naval boats that I was already used to.

We were sent to HMS *Royal Arthur*, an NCO training establishment near Winchester where we spent a lot of time on team-oriented work. This was very physical and included assault courses and a team race to carry a heavy barrel, filled with sand, across such a course. My team was not able to get the barrel to the end of the course correctly, clear of the ground, as it was so heavy.

We were sent off in groups of three on an expedition for two days and a night. We were given a number of landmarks, each of which had a numerical value, and each team had to select the route that they thought would gain them the highest score in a distance that they thought that they could cover on foot in the time available. We were provided with 24-hour ration packs and ponchos as waterproofs, but were not allowed to ask for a lift or shelter or do anything illegal.

It did of course rain and it was not a pleasant walk, in our new boots. We had by this time, as a group, become slightly more competitive and set ourselves a difficult task if we were to reach the finishing point in time. I have still got, to this day, the Ordnance Survey map with the grid references and the point values on it.

Hating rain, as I did and still do, I determined that we would not spend the night out in it and that we would find somewhere to sleep, a shed or something. In the end we found a little church that had a typical covered porch and were preparing to huddle in it when we found that the church door was not locked. We slept on the narrow wooden pews but got a better night's sleep than we might have had. We left the vicar a note telling him that we had slept there in case he wondered what had gone on.

We did well with the points and were either top or second of the teams and we got back to the rendezvous point in time. I think no one was as surprised as we were to have achieved this but the course officers were very complimentary.

These activities were done in No. 8s – Naval Working Dress – blue shirts and trousers. We had been given a cash grant to buy our No. 5 reefer suit, which I already had, and a mess kit. I simply changed my one wavy stripe for two straight stripes with red in between on my reefer jacket. I went to Goode's Brothers, on the 'Hard', to get a second-hand doeskin mess kit. Harry and Ernest were wonderful characters, Jewish brothers, who looked after you like a Lord. Optional on the clothing list was a greatcoat but the Goodes said that the raincoat, which we were issued, would be sufficient. Swords were only usually bought by career officers, but one of our intake did actually buy one. The three times that I needed a sword I borrowed one.

Harry and Ernest found me a superb second-hand mess kit, and they did the alterations to my No. 5 reefer jacket 'with their compliments'. Sadly their shop had been demolished by the time I was able to return and thank them for their kindness.

A place that we visited on the joining course was RN Prison at Lee-on-the-Solent. This was where all the 'bad boys' from the Navy, and the other services in the area, spent their time. The reason for us doctors to be there was, we discovered, that we would be responsible for the welfare of the men locked up in whatever ship or establishment we found ourselves.

Although I had had some experience of mess dinners, the others on the course experienced their first one at the Victory Barracks. The dining night was held for the leaving of the last National Service men who had opted for the three years in the Navy. It was a very riotous night that culminated in the group trying to sign their names on the ceiling of the bar. Their pyramid collapsed and the officer on the top fractured his femur.

Our intake then broke up into its professional groupings and we doctors went to the RN Medical Institute at Alverstoke. Here we learned all about the service medical record forms (F. Med's) and their specific uses. They also taught us about the medical problems specific to ships, such as galley and living space hygiene and cleanliness, together with lots of tips about treating and tracing gonorrhoea and syphilis.

Most ships in those days carried divers and we were taken to both HMS *Vernon*, the diving school, and HMS *Dolphin*, the submarine school, to learn about some of the practical problems of underwater medicine. We all had to go through the decompression chamber which was certainly an experience, although I'm not sure I would have liked to repeat it.

One night when we returned to *Victory* we found our first posting waiting for us. When I read mine at first I didn't quite understand what it meant as it read: '*Drake* additional for I.T.C.R.M. Lympstone for Commando Training.' I knew that *Drake* was in Plymouth. Someone, who I recall was hugely amused, said that ITCRM stood for Infantry Training Centre Royal Marines and that it was near Exeter. I was to join there on 13 November.

During our weeks in Portsmouth I had been up to London a few times to see Muriel. She was now sharing a basement flat in Chelsea with two other girls, Barbara and Louise. We were very much a couple again. I slept in her room and shared the sparse facilities with the others. This included an outside basement toilet. We had some good weekends and ate well in some of the well-known restaurants on the Kings Road and in the West End.

Muriel's Aunt Alice came down and she liked to eat in the Café Royal. She always drank Chateauneuf du Pape and it fell to me to taste the wine. I had to send it back as it was corked. The wine waiter obviously didn't believe me and only when the head-waiter also tried it did they agree to replace it.

I usually travelled up to London by train as it was so handy and there was not much space to park the Jaguar near the Chelsea flat. I had thought for some time that the car was too large, and not a little ostentatious, and resolved to change it. This I did on our long weekend leave before joining ITCRM.

I had had a craving for a little sports car for some time. Muriel and I went in the Jaguar to the Sports Car Centre on the Great West Road. Inside there was a row of MG TCs, about five of them, mostly 1947 onwards, in every colour except black. The salesman offered me £150 for the Jaguar, the same as I had paid for it a year earlier. We had just agreed to buy one of the cars for £150 and were about to seal the deal when into the showroom came a black one. The salesman already knew I had wanted that colour so didn't object when I said I'd have that one instead. He agreed for the same price.

What I suspect he hadn't realised was that its number plate was MG 7051, and with 19-inch bicycle wheels it was a 1946 model. We quickly swapped registration documents and left in haste lest he realised and demanded more money. We took the car up to Regent's Park, took a photograph of it, and christened it 'Maggie'. I was a bit worried about leaving it on the street in Chelsea but no harm came to it overnight.

On 12 November I drove to Exeter, in the MG, with all my goods and chattels in my 'pusser's' tin trunk strapped to the luggage carrier over the petrol tank. It was quite a long drive from London to Exeter. I arrived at Lympstone, which is just upstream of Exmouth, during the afternoon and was directed to my new accommodation.

ITCRM had just undergone major refurbishment and all the accommodation for the Marines, the NCOs and the Officers was in new three-storey blocks, all of which had lovely views over the river Exe. The Officers' Mess overlooked the main parade ground and then to the river. Everyone was thus accommodated except, that is, the Officers who were about to embark on Commando Training.

We were housed in an old brick-built block, built on the slope down from the new Officers' Mess, towards the Sick Bay at the right-hand end of the parade round. We were allowed into the Mess for our meals, but only at certain times, and we always had to change into acceptable gear before entering through the rear door only.

Three of us Officers were joining that day. John Owen, a Schoolie, an Artillery Officer and myself. None of us was fit nor previously interested in sport. We were thus aghast to learn the following morning that we had just over two weeks in which to become as fit as the rest of the squad, who had been on a 12-week basics course at Deal, who we would be joining for the Commando Course itself. These others were to turn out to be seventeen- and eighteen-year-olds! We were all in our mid twenties.

We were issued with a variety of military and camouflaged equipment including a 7.62mm self loading rifle. The standard gear was carried in two pieces of equipment; the first is worn like a waistcoat and is called fighting order and contained pouches for ammunition, mess tins, 24-hour ration pack and toilet gear. A large pack, carried on the back and resting on the back pouches of the fighting order, contained changes of clothing, socks and a large towel etc. A rolled up sleeping bag went on the top, and either a spade or a pick was strapped to its back. A poncho/ground-sheet hung from the fighting order round one's backside.

In the perverse way that only the military mind works we were not issued with the Marine DMS boots to do the course, as they were deemed too expensive to waste if we failed. We were given a second-hand pair of parade boots with steel spikes on the soles making them very slippery on smooth surfaces.

We were shown how to strip, clean and reassemble the rifle and magazines, and warned that they were expected to be clean at all times and that surprise inspections were common.

We were back into the Physical Training game with circuit, weight, rope and agility training. The idea was to try to get our legs up to marching and running long distances and our arms to hauling ourselves up, along, and over things. To start with we did this only wearing working gear but later we added the fighting order and the rifle. On our heads we wore a knitted 'comforter'.

The second morning started with a four mile road run before breakfast. The pace for these is a mixture of a fast march up hills and military doubling on the flat and downhill. The goal was for us to be able to do this in 40 minutes by the end of the two weeks. For the first few days things were sheer agony in the chest, legs and arms. By the middle of the second week we were getting more comfortable with the speed and distance, but my feet were suffering from blistering of the heels and metatarsal heads.

To strengthen our upper limbs we were introduced to the death slide, the Tarzan course, an aerial rope and wire course through trees, and the assault course which was like all other assault courses, but much worse. In addition there was the Endurance course that consisted of a series of wet and muddy obstacles and tunnels, followed by a four mile speed march back to camp. After all these physical exertions we had to fire our rifles, having been expected to have kept them clean throughout. To do this I put a condom over the end through which the first bullet would pass breaking the seal. This was immediately banned. So much for initiative.

I have to admit that I cleaned my rifle by taking it into the bath with me, the only drawback being that rust could set in, quickly, and a lot of oil had to be applied.

On the Friday of the second week we were summoned, one by one, to the Officer in Charge of Commando Training, Major Dickie Grant. He was not impressed by the state of my feet and suggested that I was back squadded and given another two weeks before I attempted the course. One reason for this is logical because if an officer fails the actual course he is sent straight back to the Navy or Army. I argued that I would either succeed in this one mammoth attempt or I would be returning to the Navy anyway and there was nothing to lose by continuing. He somewhat reluctantly agreed.

The Commando course itself started on 27 November. We were joined by Alastair Thom, another doctor, and Bill Taylor, a Padre. It is a four-week course with four tests at the end, all of which have to be passed in the same week. In our case, as Christmas intervened, we would have to take the tests in what was actually only the third week of the course, and then return after the Christmas break to do the week three coursework.

The course itself was a nightmare for me being one not interested in things physical with the next aim to do six miles in 60 minutes. The Marines are right that almost anyone can rise to a challenge and that I must have done. My view was also that they were not going to beat me, if my feet would hold out. The weather was atrocious with freezing temperatures and snow up on Dartmoor when we were up there on a load carrying exercise. We spent several nights out in it doing military exercises during which we three tended to try to keep out of the way.

We had to practise disembarking from a three ton lorry during ambush drill. My smooth-soled boots meant that I could not get a grip on the floor to get acceleration. After trying me in all positions in the lorry and each time causing the whole squad to fall in a heap either inside or outside the lorry I was put in the cab with the driver and told to stay put.

On one occasion when they sprang a rifle inspection on us there were a number of dirty rifles found by the NCOs, including our three. This earned us an extra parade one night at 1 a.m. There was freezing fog as we paraded outside the guardroom, on this occasion to be given the all clear by the NCOs. The young Lieutenant Royal Marines, our course officer who we had little time for, did not show up to inspect the rifles. We all technically outranked him and we were disgusted by his lack of courtesy. We went back to the Officers' Mess where he was asleep and woke him up with some threats of retribution if he repeated this insult.

One exercise was on Woodbury Common where we had to dig a slit trench and make it mortar proof. One of the corporals decided to make an example of my feeble attempts at this cover and made me lie in the trench, after dark, and proceeded to jump on the roof to simulate a mortar shell landing. He had been right and the roof collapsed on me. Unfortunately for both of us it trapped me rather badly with only my face showing. The weight was on my chest and legs so that I could barely breathe, and not move at all.

When he realised my predicament he had a panic attack and tore at the earth with his bare hands lest he lost a doctor on the course. His shouting brought help and after a bit of scrabbling and digging they extracted me. He was a very pale corporal who couldn't do enough to help me recover. I don't think I was really in danger, although it felt like it at the time, and it gave me a bit of pleasure to see him suffer.

The Pass Out week starts with the squad having to do nine miles in 90 minutes and finishing as a squad. The simple way to make sure the weakest get there is to put them/him in the front. The next day is the Tarzan course to be done in less than 16 minutes followed by a regain onto a wire stretched over a static water tank. Having done it correctly we Naval Officers dropped off the wire into the ice cold water while saluting smartly, to cheers from the Marines. The third day saw us on the endurance course with the four mile run back to camp in under 72 minutes, followed by firing the rifle, hitting the targets six times out of ten. I just managed all these. We then got a day off.

The fourth test is the 'Thirty Miler'. This consists of traversing Dartmoor for thirty miles carrying fighting order and rifle. It is done in groups of three; the group is not allowed to split up. We officers each had to do it with two Marines. There is a time limit on how long one takes and in the last few miles I was really struggling and my feet, especially, had had enough. I was down to slow walk and as we got near the finish and could see the lorries, I felt that we were running out of time. I ordered the two Marines to go ahead and finish. They pointed out that this was not permitted but I said that I couldn't care less if I did not stay with the Royal Marines but as it was to be their career they must finish on time, or be back squadded. They went to the finish, recorded their times and then came back and helped me, with the NCOs looking the other way. In fact I finished with 90 seconds or so to spare. In the end everyone's honour was satisfied.

At this time in my life I was as fit as I had ever been and weighed 11½ stones: three stones heavier than I had ever been before I started the course. Recovery from the ordeal, except for my feet, happened quickly, and after a bath and a sleep I set off for Christmas leave in Aberdeen in 'Maggie'. I had decided to wear my combat gear as the MG had no heater.

I drove overnight, stopping for another sleep on the way, and got to Aberdeen just after 9 a.m. Muriel and I had at long last talked about getting engaged at Christmas and when I arrived in the city I went straight to one of the jewellers on Union Street. The look of horror on the staff's faces when I entered the shop was not surprising as I was still in my combat gear and I hadn't shaved since the morning before. I hurriedly produced my ID card and apologised for my appearance. I chose three rings and surprisingly they let me take them away with me.

We got engaged that day and, as Muriel's sister Jean had also recently got engaged to Hamish, an Income Tax Inspector working in Dundee, we decided to have a double wedding in the spring. Neither I nor Hamish have been able to explain the date, 6 April, as this is the day after the tax year changes and we would lose a whole year's back tax.

I drove back to Lympstone the weekend after New Year. We had to go through the final week of training, abseiling and bouldering down near Plymouth. I had been lucky with my accident but it was nothing to the casualty rate on these two events. On the bouldering one Marine broke both wrists and another slid down a large rock taking a lot of skin off one side of his face.

I enjoyed the abseiling which we did facing down the cliff. The aim was to do the descent in two or three jumps and the show-offs would do it in one. Alistair accidently, or deliberately, tried for a single leap and it went wrong. He hit the face of the cliff, turned upside down and landed at the foot of the cliff on his head. He was unconscious and I had to abseil down to see if he was still alive. We put him in a Neil-Robertson stretcher and hauled him up the cliff. At the top he came to and seemed to be none the worse for wear.

The Friday of that week was the passing out parade and the presentation of the Green Berets. A very proud moment for everyone, but a hilarious sight with the majority of the course standing smartly to attention and being presented with their Berets with a rank of casualties behind with Marines in plasters, arms in slings and faces covered in bandages.

The Marines had all by now got postings. Alistair had been posted to 41 Commando in Aden and Bill to 40 Cdo in the Far East. I was to stay in Lympstone to give a hand in the Sick Bay, which was one doctor short.

It was a bit of a disappointment not to be going abroad but I settled down and moved into the Officers' Mess proper. I helped with sick parades and quickly found out the thinking behind making all their doctors do the course, as there were lots of attempts to get out of doing things. At the same time there were some genuine injuries and problems that the NCOs, particularly, were missing. Common ones were stress fractures and periosteitis of the tibia.

Another duty I had to do was to go up on the moor as medical cover for the long marches and the thirty miler. One evening I came off the moor and as I walked into the Mess the Senior Medical Officer offered to buy me a drink. I was surprised, and immediately suspected that there must be a reason behind this. He asked if I could get myself and my gear to Chatham by the following morning. I replied cautiously that I probably could.

If so I would be going to America. Their Lordships, in their infinite wisdom, had forgotten that to cross the Atlantic a Frigate Squadron is required to carry a doctor and that the current doctor was leaving the Navy. He, the SMO, had been authorised to ask me to go and said that the official movement order would be at the ship when I arrived.

I was delighted at the thought of a trip to America and only just managed to remember to ask when we would be returning to the UK. Mid-March was the best he could tell me. Due to get married on 6 April, I felt this was a little close, but duly rushed to phone all concerned in London and Aberdeen and then set about packing my trusty trunk again.

It snowed most of the way to Chatham. I arrived early in the morning to join HMS *Lowestoft*, a Type 12 frigate, that was to sail with the flotilla leader HMS *Berwick*. We spent two days in Chatham before sailing round to Plymouth where we ammunitioned ship, stocked up stores and refuelled for the long rough haul across the North Atlantic in January. She had a top speed of over 30 knots from her Y100 turbines but we cruised at less than half that to conserve fuel and even then we had to refuel at sea once.

On our first day at sea we went into No. 8s during the working day and I put on my Green Beret whereas all the rest were wearing blue ones. The Captain (Commander Raymond Lygo) asked if I was entitled to wear the Green Beret. When he learned that I had watch-keeping experience he said that this would be a great help if I did watches chaperoned by the senior Chief Petty Officer.

We arrived in Newport, Rhode Island after ten days during which time I had experienced severe seasickness and my assistant Leading Sick Berth Attendant Mills had had to look after me, and conduct the sick parades in my cabin.

We were warmly received by the American Navy and that first night ashore we got very merry having not had to buy a single drink. In return we hosted a party on *Lowestoft*, which was moored outside *Berwick*, and invited our hosts to see the new, and first, Bond film, *Dr No*. We had been made to promise that we would not show it in America. We didn't.

The reason for our trip was to demonstrate a new sonar and weapons system that could track their new, fast hunter-killer nuclear submarines. It depended on the two ships working together, the absence of a cone of silence under the ship and a new 3D plotting and display system, new forward firing depth charge mortars, and the speed and agility of the ships themselves.

We took on board some American Liaison Officers for our first trip to demonstrate the equipment. The skipper of the submarine became increasingly upset about being caught and eventually fell into the trap that Cdr Lygo wanted: that is, he tried to come up under us using the cone of silence. We watched him come up under us, matching our speed and we gradually increased ours to top speed, about 32 knots.

We had practised, till we were cursing, what happened next. The Y100s were thrown from full ahead to full astern in the shortest time possible without causing severe disruption to their gears. As a result the Nuclear, caught unawares, shot out in front of us and we dropped a practice mortar bomb on him.

The submarine shot off at top speed with us in hot pursuit. This chase, with *Berwick* in the lead, went on into the night. I was on the bridge, with the Chief, following *Berwick* at 32 knots at four cables. We were now closing on the Nuclear and I had awakened Cdr Lygo. He was beaten to the bridge by one of the American liaison officers who, grasping that I was in charge, was heard to say, 'Gee, shit Commander, it's the f——g doctor.'

The Nuclear had gone to the bottom of an underwater canyon. We sat on the surface above him and to get the proof that it was indeed him Cdr Lygo sent me down to the sonar paper writer that produced a tiny picture of the nuclear boat on the bottom.

A second large exercise we took part in was to provide part of the anti-submarine shield for an American aircraft carrier. LSBA Mills asked me to come and see a seaman who had developed abdominal pain. I felt that he had appendicitis. I knew that if he was no better in a few hours I would have transfer him to the carrier for possible surgery.

He got considerably worse, over the next few hours, and I had to break the bad news to the Captain. I received dire threats from both the Admiral and Cdr Lygo as to what would happen if I was wrong. It was blowing a gale and snowing and the helicopter lift was far from easy. Luckily I had been right and the surgeon on the carrier had removed a 'rotten' appendix.

We had a number of incredible parties in Norfolk and no end of offers of female companionship. The only one that took my fancy was a Portuguese girl, who had blonde hair. Her father lent me his car with written authority. I did not realise he was the Portuguese Naval Attaché.

From there we sailed back up to Bridgeport, Connecticut, and nearly created an international incident by arriving flying a large Confederate Battle Ensign that we had been given in Virginia. Our knowledge of the geography of the American Civil War had failed us.

One of the large ex-patriot community was a local General Practitioner from Scotland. He had a private plane and took me for a flight round about to show me the area. He asked if I would like to take his secretary out and said she would pick me up next lunchtime.

I was in the Wardroom, still in uniform, when the Quartermaster, with a nasty smirk on his face, announced that there was a lady at the gangway to see me. I came out on to the gangway to find the secretary in the shortest red dress that I had ever seen with, due to the wind, only partly covered black suspender belt and knickers beneath.

Almost the entire crew had by now assembled to see the 'Doctor's piece of totty' and accompanied by wolf-whistles we retreated to the Wardroom. I got her a drink and then had to leave her to the letchings of my fellow officers while I went to change. We left the ship to further wolf-whistles and drove off in her red convertible.

We set sail for home via Bermuda. We left on 1 March when there was ice on the deck as we passed New York, and it was warm and sunny when we arrived in Bermuda. We spent a few days there before the long haul home. On the way we refuelled from a French tanker and they

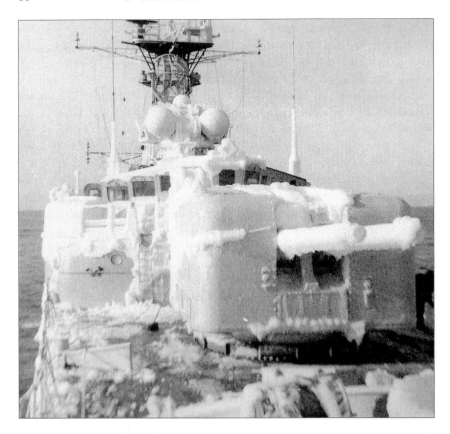

Iced-up HMS *Lowestoft*, America, 1963.

covered our deck in thick black fuel oil. We then came across a submarine and assumed it to be French. We dropped a practice grenade on her.

On our return to Chatham all the wives and sweethearts, including Muriel, had gathered to meet the ship. I went ashore to see if the MG was still in one piece. I saw her slightly to my left and as I turned in that direction fell into an open manhole. The Quartermaster had seen me go down and carried me back to the ship over his shoulder. I was a bit better the next day but covered in large bruises and was not very mobile. Thankfully the preparations for the wedding had been made while I was away.

I drove back to Lympstone where waiting for me was my long awaited posting to 40 Commando in the Far East, on 1 July. Renting seemed the only sensible solution for our accommodation and I luckily found a very small flat above the butcher's shop down in Lympstone village.

I was very delighted, and a little surprised, when the Mess presented me with an engraved cigarette box as a wedding present the day before I left to go north. I drove the MG to London and took the sleeper to Aberdeen.

My best man was John Skene, from the Charity Show days, and my usher the American Naval Medical Officer from Edzell. I forgot the wedding ring and John had to climb through the kitchen window in his morning suit while I watched, dressed in my uniform and clutching my borrowed sword. I think we were twenty minutes late at Kings College Chapel. Luckily the hairdresser took a long time with Muriel's and Jean's hair and they arrived after us! During the ceremony I got the sword caught in my shoe as I turned round and nearly fell over.

The reception was held in the Station Hotel. Hamish and I caused an immediate upset by refusing the proffered champagne and demanding a pint of beer each. Some of the relatives on Muriel's side were teetotal and there was supposed to be only orange juice on certain tables while on others the orange juice was to be laced with gin. The hotel staff got the tables the wrong way round and there was a terrible row.

Muriel and I spent the first night in the George Hotel in Edinburgh and travelled to London on the Flying Scotsman the next day, picked up Maggie the car and flew from Southend to Rotterdam. We stayed in a small hotel nearly at Arnhem. We called on Jo and Nellie in Oosterbeck who hadn't been able to come to the wedding.

On our return to Lympstone we settled into the flat and village life. Mother came down to see us and I bought her an A35 estate car that would be ideal for taking Roger the dog around. Muriel and I drove one car each back up to Aberdeen with all our possessions.

I flew out to Singapore in an RAF Comet 4. It was my first experience of flying with the RAF and I was surprised to find that the seats faced rearwards. The route took us first to El Adam in Libya, then on to Aden, Gan and the last leg, over the Indian Ocean, to Changi in Singapore. Chasing the RAF lunch menu of the day we had braised steak, with potatoes and peas, three times.

It was dark when we arrived in Singapore but even so I shall never forget the wall of humid heat that greeted us as the aircraft doors were opened. My shirt was soaking with sweat before we got to the terminal.

We were collected by a Land Rover from the Naval Base because the Unit was still at sea on HMS *Albion* on the way back from Borneo. After lunch the next day the rear party officers, wives and children gathered on the quayside with the Royal Marine Band to welcome them home.

As she got closer it became apparent that she was going too fast. The families were beginning to get a little agitated and the bandsmen could see what might be about to happen. The Bandmaster, sensing something was wrong, turned round. He immediately had the presence of mind to stop the band and then give a very clear order in a loud voice: 'Royal Marine Band and families five paces step back now.' Everyone got back to a safe distance just as *Albion* rammed into the wooden quay demolishing the first couple of feet.

I was then to witness the first of many tearful reunions. One of the Officers, realising that I was the new doctor, advised me that over seventy of the wives were pregnant, following the short Easter Leave in the middle of April, before the Unit had been sent out to Borneo. I thought he jested, but as I was to find out a few months later, he didn't.

Our base, Burma Camp, was 16 miles up into Malaya, and next to the Kota Tinggi Jungle Warfare School. The drive took us over the Causeway into Malaya, through the unforgettable sights, sounds and smells of Jahore Bahru (JB) and up the long straight road through the jungle.

This road was built by British POWs, one squad starting at JB and the other at Mersing. They were straight as a die but deliberately aimed not to meet. Eleven miles up the road, past Majedee Barracks, and the Base Vehicle Depot that held thousands of all sorts of military vehicles, there was a series of 180 degree hairpin bends joining the two ends. It claimed many Japanese drivers and their vehicles, tired from a long drive down Malaya. It continued to claim the lives of the local timber lorry drivers who often just went straight on at the first bend.

Burma Camp was the base for 40 Commando, and 145 'Miawand' Battery Royal Artillary, housing about 850 men. For my first three weeks I lived in the Mess although most of the married officers and men lived down in JB. The Colonel was John Parsons, who was remarkably like General Montgomery in many respects. I had direct access to him by simply popping my head into his Adjutant's office and saying I wanted to see the Colonel. This did not endear me to the more senior Marine Officers who did not have such easy access.

I had a staff of a Chief Petty Officer SBA, a Leading SBA Smith and 4 SBAs: Bradbeer, Bristow, Harrison and Cleary. My driver/orderly was called Millar. The first sick parade was at 0730.

While settling into the routine of the Unit I also started looking for a house. To give me some mobility I bought a Fiat 600. This had an aluminium water-cooled engine, a combination that did not go well together. Bill, the Padre who had been at Lympstone, had got a 500 which had an air-cooled engine and this seemed to work better. Mine constantly over-heated and I always had to keep a bottle of water in the car.

I found a house to rent on the outskirts of JB in Kim Teng Park. This was a large new estate built round a small hill. On the top the Chinese developer had built a row of one detached and two pairs of semi-detached houses for his family. They all seemed to crowd into the large detached one and they rented out the others.

Muriel got a flight on 21 July. We stayed in the JB Hotel on her first night. I had not known when I arrived that, once I was living in JB, I was expected to take part in either the Naval GP rota in the Naval Base, or the Army one based at Majedee. I opted for the latter but unfortunately I was put down for my first night on call that very night Muriel was due and no one would swap with me.

I got two calls that night. The first was to see to a wife who had just arrived on the same plane as Muriel, and was having hysterics when she saw a gecko on the ceiling above her head. The second was when another wife claimed that she had lost her Tampax. This was at about 2 a.m. I could not locate any Tampax then, and indeed, when examined at the Barracks next morning there wasn't one to be found.

We moved into 17, Kim Teng Park the next day. We employed an Amah called Ah Noh, who lived in the cupboard under the stairs, and inherited a black kitten called Dina, a local pye dog called Brandy and a Minah Bird who lived in the guttering.

Muriel settled in well, once she had got used to the heat. It took about ten days to become comfortable and three weeks to be fully acclimatised. The Unit was expected to have to go to Borneo in September so we decided to try to find Muriel a job. In order for her to get around we bought a second car – a convertible Ford Zephyr.

The major social gathering spot was the Officers' Club in the Naval Base. It was only a five minute drive on the Singapore side of the Causeway and we heard that there was a vacancy for a teacher in the Junior School. Muriel took this post and had to teach a variety of subjects including English, Religious Education, football and art. We were able to live on this income and my local overseas allowance, and banked my basic salary.

As well as the routine of medical care at the camp we provided daily transport to the British Military Hospital in Singapore which was 32 miles from the camp. One of the SBAs went with the patients. The Unit, like all Marine Units abroad, used a 'trickle drafting' system to change over the complement. This meant about thirty to forty new arrivals each month that had to be acclimatised and brought up to local

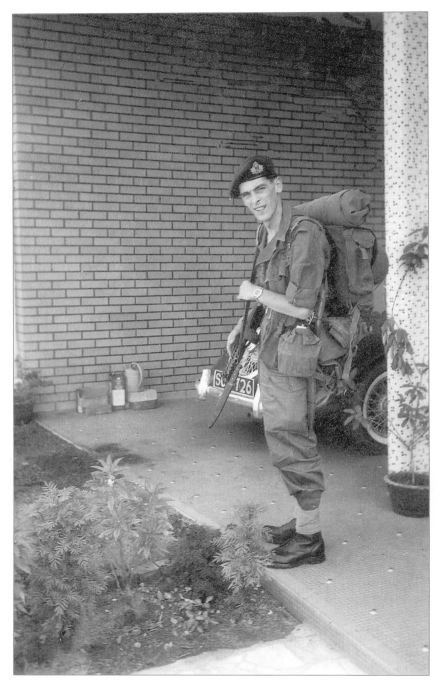

Dressed for Action, Singapore, 1963.

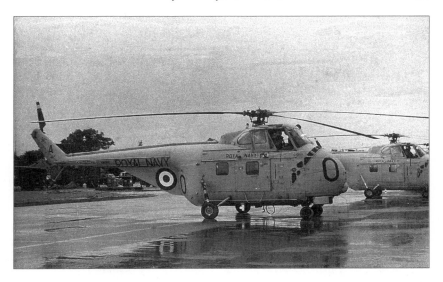

Whirlwind 7 'Oscar', Kuching, 1963.

fitness as quickly as possible. I gave many lectures on First Aid, malaria prevention, jungle hygiene and water treatment and, of course, sexually transmitted diseases which were rife in the Far East. One of our biggest orders from the stores was for condoms, which were issued free in the Navy and Marines.

The Unit was to go to Kuching, in the First Division of Sarawak, on 11 September for six months. Colonel Parsons then decided that the whole Unit was to get fit before going and gave orders that everyone, but everyone, would do a twenty-mile route march the week before. I started to get fit again and on one occasion jogged across the Causeway to the Club wearing shorts, boots and carrying an umbrella, as it was raining. Muriel went ahead in the car with my clothes but I was spotted by some astonished friends.

The 'old and bold' Marines of HQ Company were not doing very well and I came to the conclusion that if the march went ahead we were liable to be going to Borneo minus a large number of core personnel or at least with personnel not able to perform their tasks. In fear and trepidation I put this to the Adjutant who, having thought about it and seen for himself what I meant, agreed to help me put it to Colonel Parsons that he should cancel it, and he at length reluctantly agreed.

We sailed, as an intact unit, on a dreadful steamer called the SS *Auby* (nicknamed the 'Hell Ship Auby'). The light vehicles of Commando HQ were carried on deck. There was no ventilation in the ship down in the spaces that the Marines were expected to live and it was a very uncomfortable journey.

Sailing up the Kuching river to the town we disembarked and drove to Semengo Camp out at the Airport. This was a new atap-built camp placed on what, in wet weather, was obviously a swamp. The HQ stayed here and the three rifle companies were sent out to Bau, Serian and Lundu to guard the First division. Also in the camp were the Royal Irish Hussars, a cavalry unit, with Ferret, Saracen and Saladin armoured cars.

Transport was essentially by river or helicopter only. There were roads to Bau and Serian, but few further into the Division. We were served by two Naval Squadrons; 846 with Whirlwind 7s and 845 with Wessex 1s. The aircraft were still painted in their desert sand from operating in Aden. They were based on the airfield at Kuching where there was also an RAF detachment with Single and Twin Pioneers, and an Army Air Corps flight of Austers.

The temperature and humidity meant that the loads the helicopters could carry were reduced and they had to be carefully planned. They flew in pairs and they liked to have two pilots, the main problem being to spot landing sites among the 200ft trees if there was an engine failure. The Whirlwind could not lift a Land Rover so we had a number of Citroen 2cv pick-up trucks which were ideal for some of the forward bases. The Wessex could lift the cut down Land Rover, and the 105mm howitzers of the RA battery.

I had asked repeatedly that I had some helicopter drill training. I got none and sure enough a couple of days after we arrived in Borneo we got a Casevac signal which meant that I had to go out and pick up the patient. I arrived at 846 Squadron to find that I was going out with their Senior Pilot, a Marine Captain. I explained to the ground crew that I had no experience of flying operationally. They handed me a hammer and a set of jump leads, opened the engine door covers and showed me where to hit the 'likely to jam' cartridge start mechanism and where to attach the jump leads. The spare battery was already in the cabin where they strapped me into the crewman's place and wished me luck.

The flight time to most of our outposts was thirty minutes or more, and I felt very lonely all that time not able to talk to the pilot. We picked up the casualty and returned in one piece. I spent most of every day after that touring our various bases doing sick parades, as well as any extra flights from Casevac requests. The squadron presented me with proper flying gear and headset, so that I could communicate with the pilots. Thereafter I usually flew up front, wherever possible, learning to fly.

These routine visits to the three Company HQs, with their own SBA, and to the more isolated troop locations, plus the knowledge among the Marines that 'their doc' would come and get them if anything happened to them, did wonders for the esteem of the whole of the sick bay staff.

Bau had been a centre for gold mining in the past and the first time I flew in I was amazed at the deep blue colour of the local lake; it was full of 'Royals' swimming. The pilot explained that this colour was due to the cyanide that had been used to extract the gold. Luckily by the time I got it put out of bounds no one had swallowed sufficient to be ill.

In our fiercest military encounter of the tour we picked up the trail of a full company of enemy coming down from the border. The Colonel set in motion plans to stop them short of Bau and ordered me there with the Regimental Aid Post. I was not happy about this as it meant that after dark I would cut off from the rest of the Unit. He was adamant and I went. I, however, was right and the engagement took place away from Bau and I had to be moved back to Kuching at high speed in the dark, without lights, and with an escort of armoured cars.

In the engagement a half section of our Marines, under a Lance Corporal (five men), came across a full company of enemy (100). In an incredible action they stopped and then turned the enemy although nearly running out of ammunition. Regretfully the Lance Corporal was killed and one of the Marines slightly injured. We were all very proud when he was later awarded the Posthumous Military Medal.

The next day I flew out and was involved in the follow-up operation. From the bloodstains it was evident that our patrol had caused them a number of severe casualties, all of whom had been carried away. All their equipment had been abandoned in their haste to get back across the border.

In the north, at Lundu, there was, at that time, the world's biggest bauxite mine. Although there was no oil in the first division there was coal in large quantities in the hills but although the natives burnt it they didn't really see it of any value to mine commercially.

We had a company of attached Gurkhas, and a Gurkha signals detachment. Their ambushes seemed very successful and they captured a few infiltrators but at the same time sustained one or two casualties.

The worst injury was a chest wound sustained during an ambush. I collected him at dawn and put a chest drain in but even with that in place he would stop breathing before we could clear the 200ft trees. The pilot was the CO of 845 squadron, 'Tank Sherman'. We got him back to Kuching by picking our way through the trees. We had radioed ahead that he would need to be got to Singapore and they held a Hastings for him.

I explained to the pilot that we could not get him above 200ft and as the Hastings was not pressurised they would need to be careful. They got him there safely and he too survived. I met the pilot a few weeks later and asked him how he had got on with the breathing problem. He astonished me by saying that he simply kept the plane below 200ft all the way and that he hadn't had so much fun since he had been on the Dam Buster Raid.

The Unit was under command of 3 Cdo Brigade HQ based in Kuching town. The Brigade Medical Officer, David Mends, and I did not hit it off and he did not really agree with the way in which I ran the Medical cover, particularly my willingness to let the SBAs have more responsibility than normal. On a number of occasions he openly criticised the way cases had been handled and on one occasion took out all the stitches one of the SBAs had very carefully and neatly put in.

We had many military and political visitors, some less welcome than others. The Duke of Edinburgh spent a day with us and helicoptered around a number of our border locations. I was introduced to him at the airport. I then flew ahead of him to each LZ. At the third he said, 'We'll have to stop meeting like this – Doc.' I found him pleasant, charming and very human.

The two Navy squadrons were recalled to the Carriers and were replaced by 225 Sqdn (Whirlwind 10s) and 22 Sqdn (Belvederes) of the RAF. 225 had been the original tri-service experimental helicopter unit and their tie still depicted this. They brought an RAF doctor with them who announced that he would do all the Casevac-ing and would have priority call on aircraft over me. This lasted a couple of days after which he decided it was too dangerous spending so much time over the jungle and that I could go back to doing it. This was just as well as the Marines were working themselves up to complain.

The very next morning we got a Casevac call at dawn to one of the furthest outposts. I got up to the airfield to find that the CO of 225 Squadron was taking me and he invited me into the cockpit. After we had taken off, and I was plugged in to talk to him, he said that he understood that I could fly these aircraft. I admitted that I could, a bit, and he asked where were we going. I pointed to a large solitary tree about twenty miles away and said, 'we turn left there.' 'You seem to know where we're going, doc; you'd better take us there.' Which I did and our relationship with 225 became as it had been with the Naval squadrons.

22 Sqdn was more aloof because they always flew with two pilots anyway. The Belvedere, I felt, was a highly dangerous aircraft with two engines which flew squint which became obvious when there was a patient with an IV drip up which didn't hang vertical to the fuselage. The Twin Pioneer was deemed so dangerous that even the RAF advised me not to travel in one if avoidable. I took them up on the advice and never did.

One afternoon we received a message that one of the Army Air Corps Austers, on a mail run and with a visiting RAF padre on a 'jolly', on board, had been shot down near the border. One of our patrols had seen it crash and was on the way to the scene. I was briefed by the Colonel himself and, as there was only one chopper available, I would have to go without an escort. I took an SBA, a hamper of supplies and stretchers. As I was leaving the Ops room the Colonel asked me to radio back any military information to him to help catch the perpetrators.

Leaving the ops room I met a Gurkha signaller and I told him to stay there till things quietened down a bit. We dashed off and approached the site of the crash, a helicopter Landing Zone, at about 4000 ft in case the enemy were still around looking for a second target. We could see the wreckage, which looked almost intact at one end of the LZ, and troops around it. The radio confirmed that it was our patrol; the Padre was dead but the pilot alive, although injured. We radioed this news back to Kuching then did a vertical drop, auto-rotating, into the LZ.

The Padre had been shot in the reverse direction through the spine to Lord Nelson. The pilot's right arm had been broken by another bullet through the humerus and he had crash-landed the plane in this helicopter LZ using his knees to control the joystick and his remaining arm to work the flaps and throttle. The plane was nearly intact as he had managed to stall it in.

It was getting dark by now and so we decided, having splinted his arm and started a drip, to fly the pilot out while we could, leaving the Padre with the patrol to return for him the next day. We flew back in the dark, not something that was encouraged in those days because of the lack of instrumentation, but once airborne the lights of Kuching guided us home. This was only our second fatality from enemy action and reinforced the view that 'jollies' were potentially dangerous.

The Gurkha with the message was still standing outside the ops room and smartly came to attention as I approached, saluted and asked me if it was quiet enough to pass his message now. I replied that I would check, popped my head in and came out to him and said it was. Luckily it wasn't an important piece of information but I was suitably embarrassed.

The Marines' appetite for the opposite sex was unlimited and although Kuching market was out of bounds, because someone threw a grenade into it, there were plenty of other places to go. They even tried to smuggle girls back into the camp in the back of the trucks. One night, in November I was awoken in the middle of the night to be told of a case of suspected buggery in one of the huts. This was a serious offence, certainly in those days, and I had to take samples from various places and send them, and clothing, off for forensic examination. Nothing conclusive came of this.

Also in November, and into December, the babies conceived in April arrived. I am glad I was not in JB or Singapore at the time as the whole

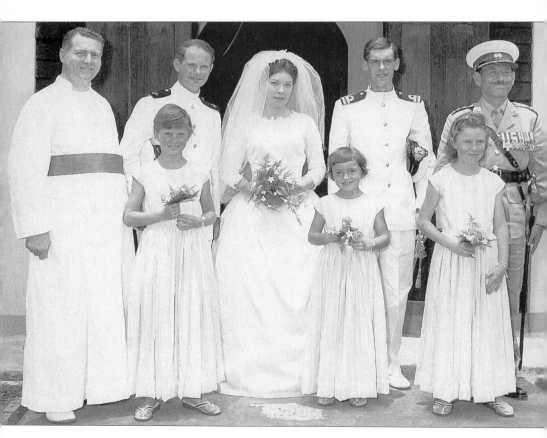

Bill the Padre's wedding.

maternity system and BMH were overwhelmed with up to six being born each day during a single week.

It was strange to spend Christmas in Kuching. It was when entertaining local ex-patriots and sipping afternoon tea that a long burst of machine-gun fire went though the Mess. Before anyone could move another one followed it and everyone threw themselves on the floor. There was a terrible crash of breaking china in the silence that followed.

Some of us sensed that it had come from inside the camp and ran round to where a fitter was working on an armoured car and was just about to try, for the third time, to replace the machine gun in the turret of a Ferret. This is fired by a foot trigger and he had had his foot on it while lowering the gun into place.

We returned to Singapore on 1 February 1964 where we spent three months reorganising and retraining. The Zephyr had shown it could be very dangerous due to an insoluble brake problem and we traded it in for a black MG TF. I helped to deliver a baby at home who I then had to rush to the medical centre on its father's knee in the MG. I learned how easy it is to get the sex wrong as at birth I was certain it was a boy, but it turned out to be a girl.

We went to two weddings in both of which Muriel was 'the bride's mother'. The first was Graham Reid to Wendy, and the second was Bill, our Padre, to Freda. I was Bill's best man but my speech upset his parents who had not met me before.

One of the biggest worries of the military planners was that the enemy might try, and succeed, to capture one of the vital airfields in Borneo and it was up to the Marine unit, not in Borneo, to recapture it. We had to practise this and sailed in *Bulwark* from 4 to 8 May up the coast of Malaya where we practised an amphibious assault.

The day after we returned after these three and a half weeks at sea I was summoned 'at once' to the Naval Base. I went as I was in Marine shirt, shorts and belt, and green beret. I was ushered in to this large room full of some very senior naval officers, all in whites. I was immediately asked why I was wearing khaki and told off for hazarding security. I was none too pleased at this telling off.

The assembled officers then proceeded to discuss, in great detail, what was obviously meant to be a highly classified proposal. I raised my arm to point out that I wasn't sure that my security classification was high enough for this. After a whispered conversation at the other end of the table a typed copy of a declaration of the Official Secrets Act was placed in front of me to sign.

All this led to me being absent from home for another ten days, a near divorce, a near court martial for losing my Dangerous Drugs, a great deal of excitement and the smallest part of an MBE.

The Americans were becoming more and more involved in Vietnam during this time and in May we set off again in *Bulwark* to the Philippines where we spent a few days in Subic Bay. The assembled fleet was possibly the largest assembled since D-Day and included at least five aircraft carriers. Getting back from shore, to the many ships of many nationalities, was a nightmare and there were queues of sailors and Marines waiting for boats. The American MPs had little understanding of man management except brute force, and on one occasion when things were getting ugly we Officers ordered our Marines to come round and use our jetty.

In early June the whole fleet took part in a huge amphibious landing on one of the islands in an exercise called 'Ligtas'. It was very hard work and we were on the go constantly for several days but 'Royal', as usual, excelled himself and won much praise from the Americans. It was during this trip, sitting on the flight deck, that I realised that my longterm career would have to involve some form of surgery.

A month later the Unit sailed for its next tour of duty, in north Borneo. On this occasion we travelled in *Sir Lancelot*, a Landing Ship Logistics (LSL) which had a Royal Fleet Auxiliary crew. For us Officers the trip was comfortable in the accommodation in the superstructure but the Marines had another very uncomfortable one in the mess-decks.

We were based right round the top of Borneo, near Tawau, in an area very close to the border with Indonesia which had previously been garrisoned by Malay troops, and then Gurkhas. Commando HQ was at Kalabakan, a logging centre forty miles away, and one which the Indonesians had attacked and nearly overrun when Malay troops had been there a few weeks previously. Expecting them to come back and try again the Malays had been cleverly replaced by Gurkhas. The Indonesians did re-attack and got a nasty surprise. They were driven off with some loss to themselves.

The logging company belonged to the Bombay-Burma Company and was managed by a Dutchman called Huck and his wife Honey. They had a beautiful bungalow with a swimming pool and games room with a snooker table and bar. They let us, the Naval Officers, use these and it was here that I, together with Bill the Padre and John the Schoolie, grew our first beards. Mine grew in ginger, my Celtic ancestry I presume. Having seen the Officers growing, all my sick bay staff followed suit. It had a very interesting effect in that the locals, most of whom can't grow beards, were terrified of us.

The crossing point for the Kalabakan incursion was an old shop at Serudong Laut where we stationed B Coy. Two weeks later Bradbeer, the SBA, reported that he had a number of cases of what he thought, from the books, was Dengue Fever. We had been confidently told that the one tropical disease that did not occur in north Borneo was Dengue. All indications were that we did indeed have it so I set Bradbeer the epidemiological task of finding the vector. A few days later an envelope arrived from him with a (dead) small black and white striped mosquito: the vector Aedes Aegypti.

The fever was debilitating, but self-limiting. Because of the logistical problem of Casevac-ing everyone who got it we nursed them there by setting up a small in-patient facility and naming it 'The Royal Naval Hospital Serudong Laut'. At the same time we set about eradicating the vector by spraying as it has a fairly limited flying range. No visitors were allowed to stay the night there unless for a vital reason.

No one in our Command, or Singapore, believed us nor was the slightest bit interested so I turned to the Americans and used one of the contacts I had made on 'Ligtas'. He advised me that there was a Tropical Diseases Unit in Kuala Lumpur which I contacted and we sent samples of blood to them. They confirmed that we did indeed have Dengue Fever.

A few weeks later the cases dried up and we had no more new ones while we were there. I wrote the incident up with all the blood results provided by the Americans and it was published in the *Journal of the Royal Naval Medical Service* (the 'Guffer's Gazette') in 1973.

Supply, and one reserve Company, remained on a rubber plantation near Tawau, called Bombali. This company was split up into Troops, and even Sections, and stationed in land bases, and on boats, along the sea and river border with Indonesia. With the Unit so spread out there was again a great deal of flying to be done as I moved round all these locations regularly. Initially we again had 846 Sqn, with their Whirlwind 7s, but as they were very limited in their carrying capability they were reinforced by a flight of 225 Sqn RAF's Whirlwind 10s.

In this part of Borneo there were a number of airstrips which could take small planes and we had a single Army Air Corps Beaver with a single Sergeant pilot based at Tawau. He also discovered that I had some experience in flying and so set about teaching me to be the co-pilot to him on our many trips together.

I had two memorable events on this aircraft. The first was on a trip from Tawau to Kalabakan with me flying the plane. We had a full load of passengers including one of our senior NCOs. There came a tap on my shoulder and I was handed a note from this NCO which read, 'You wouldn't like me to take out your appendix and I don't like you flying this f——g plane.'

The second occurred as we were taking off from a short strip, with one of our officers in the back; the cockpit filled with blue smoke. The Sergeant shut the throttle and stamped on the brakes but as the strip was very short he did a ground loop so we came to rest facing the other way at the edge of the water. He and I tumbled out either side lest it burst into flames, forgetting Jasper in the back. The smoke cleared to reveal Jasper still struggling to climb out and cursing us more and more as we, by this time, were seeing the funny side of it.

846 Sqn was again recalled to the Carrier and was replaced by a Malay Air Force squadron of Alouette 3s. These are French built aircraft and while able to carry five passengers did not have the freight capacity of the Whirlwinds. We felt lucky that their maintainence, while we were there, was done by a detachment of the New Zealand Air Force whose supply aircraft was a Bristol 'Frightener'.

The night before 846 Sqn flew back to the Carrier we had a monumental party in their mess as they said that they were not going to take any of their remaining alcohol supply back to the ship. We sat up all night playing poker to achieve that goal. I asked, early in the evening, what they were going to do with their three gas powered fridges. (We did not have any in the mess at Kalabakan.) The CO agreed to sell them all to me for 100 Malay Dollars (about £12). I paid for them by

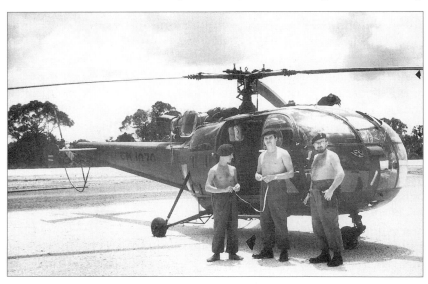

Alouette 3 and 'Team' Kalabakan, North Borneo, 1964.

signing a bar chit, hoping I would be reimbursed, and wrote on it 'including delivery'.

I flew back in the Beaver the next day with a dreadful headache and retired to bed after lunch to be awoken by the sound of a Whirlwind followed by a request from the airstrip as to where I wanted these fridges. The CO of the squadron had flown them up himself. I got my 100 dollars back from the mess treasurer and we sold them on to the Unit that replaced us at a profit.

The Unit gained another decoration in the form of a Military Cross. I was present on that occasion and recall that most of my medicinal brandy was consumed, not by the combatants but by the nervous medical staff and senior officers present. The decorated officer was wounded in the arm but required only scant attention, and a sling, from me.

In the middle of December we were replaced by 42 Cdo, the exchange being done by helicopters of 845 Sqn from *Bulwark* which anchored off to do the exchange. By the time it was my turn to fly to the carrier it was dusk and we were to be the last flight of the day. When we landed, in the dark, the pilot let down with his tailwheel over the edge of the flight deck. I could see this as I was sitting in the crewman's seat at the door. I was able to speak to him and I shouted a warning but made to jump out into the water (many feet below) when he yanked back on the collective and we shot up into the air again with me sharply pulled by gravity back into my seat; luckily.

There followed a pleasant five-day passage on the ship back to Singapore where the families were eagerly awaiting us. Included was my mother who had flown out to be with us for two months over Christmas and New Year. We had a busy time showing Mother round as much as we could. She really enjoyed herself and even got into the local Singapore newspaper when she reported one of the sales assistants in Tang's store for trying to diddle her.

The night before she was due to fly home, 17 February, she said that she was feeling tired, had got heartburn and went to bed early. A short time later she woke us to say the heartburn was getting worse and it was obvious to me that she was having a heart attack. We called an ambulance from Majedee and took her down to BMH Singapore. By this time it was apparent that she was very unwell, was grey and still in great pain in spite of morphine given before we set off.

An ECG confirmed that she had had a massive infarct and she lapsed into unconsciousness. The Consultant Physician, who by now had seen her, told me that it was a non-survivable infarct, and indeed Mother died before dawn.

We decided that, as she had had such an enjoyable time in Singapore, we would request that she be buried in the Ulu Pandan Military Cemetery. Permission was granted and the funeral was held there. A headstone was carved with the following inscription by Shelley: 'Death is the veil which those who live call life: They sleep, and it is lifted.'

I took compassionate leave after the funeral to fly home to settle Mother's affairs in Aberdeen. Muriel and I had decided that if we were to return to the United Kingdom we would need a base of our own so decided to keep No. 60, and rent it for the next eight months while we were still in Singapore. We were lucky, or so we thought at the time, to hear of a Bank Manager who wanted to rent until the autumn.

I took the opportunity whilst in UK to go and discuss my possible future postings if I extended my Commission in the Navy. I got to the office as directed but there was no one there. A file, with my name on it, was on the desk. It was empty except for my joining papers. We discussed the possibility of me staying on and going to one of the Naval Hospitals for a spell. There was no commitment forthcoming about the possibility of my being put into a surgical training programme. I received a letter in Singapore offering me such a post in Plymouth, but I would need to transfer to the Permanent List.

My flight back to Singapore was the cause of my refusing to fly as a passenger again for many years. On this occasion the plane was an Eagle Airways Britannia. I had flown in them before and they were very quiet and comfortable planes. We staged through Bombay and on take-off, in the dark, we suddenly lost power. We then lost even more power and started going sideways. I recall passing Bombay railway station level with its clock and then we were out over the bay where the water, black and illuminated by the street lights, was not very far below. Knowing a little about flying I reasoned that we had lost both port engines but this alone did not fully explain our predicament as a Britannia is capable of functioning on only two engines.

We flew like this for another fifteen minutes while the Captain dumped fuel and agonisingly slowly we began to climb. About half an hour after take-off the Officers on board, about four of us, were summoned forward to be briefed on the situation. The good news was that the Senior Training Captain was also on board doing a flight check on the crew. The bad news was that the 'extra' that I had suspected was that there had been a hydraulic failure as well and the port undercarriage leg was still down while the other two were up.

We were to prepare for a ditching, although this did not seem a good option with the port gear down. We made an agonisingly slow flat turn back towards Bombay where we were given a straight in approach. The Captain had explained that he didn't know what would happen when he tried to lower the rest of the undercarriage. In the event it went down but he had no means of telling if it had locked or not. The touch down, when it came, was one of the smoothest I have ever experienced in my life; and the undercarriage held up.

The following three months were spent in a rather boring routine which is very bad for the young Royal Marine as it leads to all sorts of disciplinary problems. By June we all felt we needed to take the Unit back on active service. The wives of course were not of the same opinion.

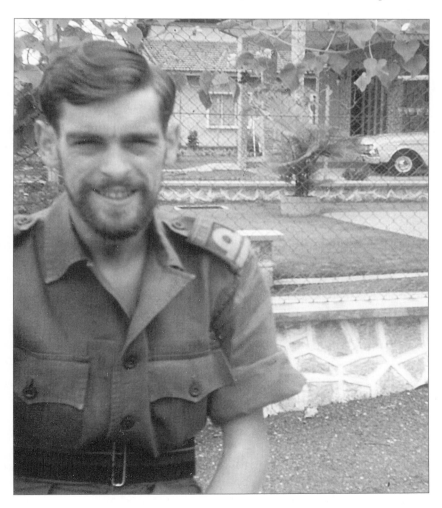

My first beard, 1965.

We returned to the first division of Sarawak but were all based at Serian where we had had only a Company last time. The Indonesian Regulars had just given 2 Para a hard time at Plaman Mapu, having got through the wire and into one of the mortar pits, before being driven out. There was a feeling that there would continue to be such raids along that part of the border but in fact nothing very much materialised during the three months I was there.

Helicopter support was again provided by Whirlwind 10s and Belvederes but by this time we had received three Bell 49Gs of our own. In addition land transport was a lot easier round Serian as there were one or two rudimentary roads.

We were now under command of the Army's 99 Brigade and one day I was summoned to meet the Colonel in charge of the Medical Unit. I drove to Kuching and as we were on active service I was carrying my usual assortment of weapons, which were needed in case of an ambush. These included my Stirling sub-machine gun with three magazines taped back to back, my 9mm Browning in its holster and two smoke grenades, one hanging from each 'D' ring on the front of my fighting order. I was in jungle greens and boots, with a Royal Marine belt, Green Beret and my camouflaged naval epaulettes all covered in a fine layer of dust.

I stood in front of his desk and saluted with my Stirling at my side. He looked me up and down for a long time and then all he said was, 'Why aren't you wearing your Sam Brown?' I realised in an instant that I was likely to waste my time trying a long explanation and simply replied, 'Naval Officers do not wear Sam Browns, Sir.' He looked intently at my epaulettes and then gave me a lecture about soldiering, not to get into his bad books, and then I was dismissed.

His Adjutant then tried to issue me with a 3 ton white ambulance with red crosses all over it. I attempted to explain that the enemy tended to use the red crosses for target practice and anyway we were Special Forces not covered by the Geneva Convention. He was also clearly bemused and said to please myself about the ambulance. A few weeks later one of those ambulances was indeed ambushed and badly shot up along one of the roads.

I left Borneo on 21 August 1965 on a Comet of Malaysian Airways for Singapore at a cost of £15. I do not remember very much about the trip as my Officer colleagues had dined me out in Serian the night before and had been plying me with drink all that day before handing me over to two gorgeous stewardesses who looked after me handsomely on the flight. They almost had to carry me down the steps of the plane in

Singapore and I can still see the look on Muriel's face as I descended the steps with an arm round each of these beauties.

The incident in Bombay had put me off flying so we booked to sail home on MV *Victoria* of the Lloyd Triestino line. We sailed from Singapore straight to Jakarta where I spent the day keeping out of sight of the armed Military Policeman on the gangway. Then we called at Bombay just as India and Pakistan were squaring up for a war over Kashmir, and then on to Karachi when the war started in earnest that very day. I was not impressed with either city, particularly with the organised begging by mutilated children, and have never had any desire to pay to go back to either of those countries.

Aden being still too dangerous we called at Djibouti, in French Africa, opposite. This was a fascinating place and we found a bar that was just like Rick's bar in 'Casablanca' with all the trimmings, including a piano player. Our last call was Egypt as we passed through the Suez Canal. We visited Cairo and Alexandria but while interesting to see I would again not wish to repeat it. The last leg was across the Med and up the Adriatic to Venice where we spent a long weekend seeing the sights before travelling back to UK by train.

I was technically released from the Navy on 2 September but got a month's extra pay in lieu of terminal leave. I enquired what my next posting was to be if I signed on. I was only slightly surprised to be told that I would be going to The Liverpool School of Tropical Medicine and Hygiene to do the DTM&H, after which I would be going back to the Far East for another tour as Brigade Medical Officer, with advanced promotion to Lieutenant Commander. I thanked them kindly and resolved to try my hand at surgery in the National Health Service.

CHAPTER ELEVEN

Early Surgical Training: Aberdeen, 1966–1968

O N OUR ARRIVAL back in the United Kingdom, at Victoria Station, we went straight to Slough to collect our new car which we had ordered from Singapore. We had chosen a blue Saab Sport. It was our first new car, cost £899 and had the registration number LBH656C.

We stayed with Muriel's parents at Queens Road, while we sorted out No. 60. It cost us almost all the income we had received from the Bank Manager, in rent, to redecorate and put it back into reasonable shape. We moved back in and retrieved Roger who had been with friends in the country since Mother left to visit us in Singapore.

I immediately set about getting myself back into the Health Service, and surgery. The first thing I did was to shave off my beard as they were still frowned upon in surgery, believed to harbour bacteria. I arranged an appointment to see George Smith, the new Professor of Surgery. He had my University exam results on his desk and noted that most of my marks had been mediocre and wanted to know why I wanted to take up surgery starting, as I was, three years behind my contemporaries. The only thing in my favour seemed to be that I had got Distinction both in Anatomy and Surgery in my undergraduate days.

He agreed to help me but pointed out that, as I had done a pure Orthopaedic House Job, I would need to do at least three months' General Surgery, at this level, to satisfy the conditions for the Primary FRCS exam. I was lucky in that Stracathro came to my rescue and Mr Clarke was able to give me the three months I needed from 1 February 1966.

Muriel decided to do a Diploma in Education starting in October. She preferred to do this rather than the teacher training course so that she was well qualified to get a better teaching post in the long run, if she wished. There was no sign of Muriel becoming pregnant and as we had never used any form of contraception we were a little surprised, and beginning to become a little concerned.

To earn some money in the meantime I managed to get a two months locum post, in November and December, as Senior House Officer in Physical Medicine (now more commonly known as Rheumatology) at the City Hospital which was down near the sea front. Needing two cars again I put Maggie (now nearly twenty years old) back on the road and went to work every day in her. It snowed early that winter and I was viewed as something of a crank arriving in the MG in the snow.

I went off to Stracathro at the end of January 1966. It was a little galling to be only a Houseman again but I was realistic enough to realise it just had to be done. I also had to go back to being on call on a 1 in 2 rota which I was to continue for many years.

I started my surgical training proper at Forresterhill on 1 May 1966. My first three months were in the Professorial Unit. I found that the new Professor and Norman Matheson, Senior Lecturer, did not get on at all and fought over the use of beds.

Aberdeen was, in those days, at the forefront of renal transplantation that was in its infancy. One of my jobs was to sit with the patients on dialysis for hours, mainly at night. The machinery then was a huge thing like an upright tub washing machine called a Kolft Dialiser. It was in the days long before Aids had been heard of and the tubing carrying the blood from the patient to the machine, and back again, would sometimes burst, owing to pressure, covering everything in blood. We had to apply large clamps to the ends of the ruptured tubing before the patient, and the machine, became ex-sanguinated. Sharing this boring task with me was a Norwegian called Jetmund Engeset. He is still there, as Senior Lecturer, and he and I are now in the same Surgical Travelling Club.

On 1 August I moved Units to where the senior Surgeons were Norman Logie and Sidney Davidson. They were of the old school and expected the best from you at all times. Mr Davison particularly was a bit of a tyrant and insisted in counter-signing all your letters before he would allow them to go out of his department. He used a proper ink pen to alter letters, in longhand, which were then retyped.

The work, although hard, instilled great surgical discipline which in many respects was no different from the Military sort. In theory it was a 1 in 2 rota but in reality it was more than that as we had to be there every Saturday morning for a ward round, and we only had one Sunday a fortnight completely off. It was difficult to do simple things like get a haircut, or get to the bank.

The younger surgeons – in those days Scotland still had Senior and Junior Consultants – were James Kyle, David Blair and Andrew Foote. Much of my early learning in surgical skills was from these three together with their senior registrars John Steyn and Alan Davidson. In those days learning surgery was very much an apprenticeship system with the trainee being allowed to do the next level of complexity of operation once satisfying his mentors of his capabilities.

I had always been good with my hands so that once shown an operation, and having understood the anatomy of the field, I could usually do it. My operating skills soon far outreached my theoretical knowledge required for the first part of the FRCS that I would have to get as soon as possible. This was, and maybe still is, the most difficult exam for a trainee surgeon to have to pass. It consists of Anatomy (unchangeable), Physiology (always seeming to be changing) and Bio-chemistry (seemingly in its infancy and changing daily). The latter two subjects had changed so much in the seven years since I had done them that I basically had to start again at square one.

On 'take' nights it was quite usual to receive twenty emergency cases and frequently we would finish the night with beds down the middle of the Nightingale wards. These were no problem and mostly disappeared by the next lunchtime. It did ensure that all our patients were in one place and therefore were much better supervised than if spread out all over the hospital in all sorts of wards. In those days you were responsible for your own consultant's cases at all times.

Muriel got her Diploma in Education and then a job at Summerhill School starting in the autumn. By the end of 1966 I had convinced most of my seniors of my clinical acumen and surgical skills. Studying proved hard and I realised that I was going to have to take six months out to do a full-time course in the Basic Sciences in the London College, and live in the Nuffield College next door.

I was on call over New Year. On 2 January a man appeared in the ward. He had abdominal pain and wanted a 'mixture' for it. He had awoken that morning after his Hogmanay celebrations with this pain. He had to go to theatre for a perforated duodenal ulcer to be repaired and all his New Year alcohol recycled through the drains. The following morning he took his own discharge. Sister reminded him, as she tried to stop him, that he had stitches in and that they would need to be removed in about ten days. Expecting him back the next day we were proved wrong. On the 10th day, however, he reappeared and asked Sister to remove the stitches.

I started the Primary course in London on 1 February 1967. Anatomy was taught by Professor Last who had written a very good, but different and contentious, textbook. I stuck to Lockhart and this did not endear me to him. His assistant was Dr Stansfield, who was a wonderful teacher, and who liked to have a beer with 'the boys'.

On the course there were a number of us who were older than others. I became particularly friendly with two and we went out for a drink just before closing time, which was 10.30 in those days. One was Tony Revell, later Medical Director General of the Navy, who was studying to be an anaesthetist, and the other a South African called Roger who had been involved in the war in Biafra as a medical mercenary.

One night as we were returning to the college the first was followed by a 'ruffian'. On the Underground platform the 'ruffian' accosted our friend. Roger went to one side and I the other of the 'ruffian'; we leant him back over the rails (there was no train approaching). This was the first time that I witnessed that a non-Caucasian can go pale. We asked him to apologise, which he did with alacrity, and we let him go.

I joined two Clubs. One was the Playboy Club which had pleasant bars, pleasant 'Bunny' waitresses, good steak sandwiches and live music and entertainment. Dudley Moore and his Quartet played there frequently and I saw Dave Allan several times. The second was the 'Tatty Bogle' that was in a rather seedy back alley in Soho but was a very good Jazz Club.

At the end of the course, in May, I sat the Primary exam. I knew that I did not know enough to pass and sure enough I didn't. I then studied hard for the next attempt at the exam in Edinburgh in June. I knew a lot more by then and felt more confident about the style of the exam. I failed again but this time by a much smaller margin. I resolved to keep trying in the short term and at least until I had done my next required job. If I had not succeeded by then I would have to return to the Navy.

Muriel had still not become pregnant, in spite of determined efforts and careful planning. We decided to find out why and Muriel went through all the tests and was given a clean bill of health. We then discovered that my live sperm count was very low. While fertility was not entirely ruled out it was deemed unlikely. We immediately decided to set about adopting and were accepted onto the books of the Scottish Adoption Society in Edinburgh.

An aim of mine, having crossed the Equator in the Navy, had been to go to the Arctic Circle and see the midnight sun. We took the Saab Sport to Helsinki and stayed in the posh Helsinki Hotel for two nights. Muriel wanted a sauna that was on the top floor of the hotel. After she had had the heat room and the massage, she was ushered naked through a door by a 'Brunhilda type' attendant, who did not speak English, on to the roof of the hotel in full view of anyone watching.

St Petersburg (Leningrad as it still was then) was only a few miles away and so we set off to see if we could get into Russia to see the palaces. Only when I was in sight of the border did I remember that I was not allowed to enter the Soviet Union by the terms of my service with the Navy.

We drove north through the forest parallel to the Russian border and camped at the side of a huge lake near the town of Kuopio, which is roughly half way to the Arctic Circle. The next day we set off for Rovaniemi, on the Arctic Circle. It is about 250 miles further north and we needed petrol. There were few garages marked on the map and we nearly missed the only one on our road as it was up a side road, on the opposite side to that depicted on the map, and I just saw it in time.

We were booked into the Rovaniemi Motel, a log cabin motel. All our hotels had been prepaid through Thomas Cook and we were carrying vouchers. I presented the voucher and the response was, 'Who are Thomas Cook's?' They eventually phoned someone in Helsinki before being satisfied that we had paid.

We only stayed there the one night to experience the almost 24 hours of daylight and then turned south again through Sweden to Norway where we camped beside a frozen lake just outside Trondheim before making for Bergen, and the ferry back to Newcastle. We arrived tired and thirsty at the booked hotel in Bergen and having dumped our bags, and before having a shower, asked where the bar was to be told that we had been booked into a temperance hotel.

I had arranged to do the next requirement for surgical training which is six months in Casualty at Woolmanhill, in the centre of the city, on 1 August 1967. The Consultant in Charge was David Proctor and he had an assistant, Charlie Burroughs, who had trained to be an Orthopaedic Surgeon. The department was an exceedingly busy one dealing with trauma, simple fractures, medical emergencies and a host of attempts at suicide.

I decided to do a little research into the possible reasons behind the suicide attempts. Many of the patients simply said that they had become very depressed and I wondered if there was any connection between their depressions and atmospheric depressions. I charted the daily numbers of these episodes and there certainly were small peaks. I then rang Dyce Airport weather centre and asked them for the daily pressures.

The result was interesting in that there was a correlation between troughs of low pressure and the peaks for suicide attempts which were on the day after the atmospheric low. No one was interested in publishing this finding then but the condition called Seasonally Affected Disorder (SAD) is now a well recognised phenomenon.

The news came suddenly that the Adoption Society had a baby to offer us, born on Friday 13 October, in Edinburgh. We of course jumped at the chance and had a frantic few days buying all the necessaries that most couples have nine months to do. We drove down and collected James Robert when he was only a week old. Muriel had had to pack in her job quickly but the school had been very understanding. The omens must have been good because I also passed the primary in Glasgow the following week on the 27th.

I saw an advertisement for a Jaguar XK150 coupé in the local evening newspaper. On the floor beside the car was a spare engine and it emerged that this was the original Blue Spot engine, half way between the standard car engine and the 'S' which had three carburettors. The engine in the car was a standard 3.4L Jaguar engine. I made an offer for the car, plus the extra engine, and this was accepted.

I worked on the original engine and although big they are relatively simple mechanically. I got all the spares I needed from the local Jaguar agent who thought I was quite crazy to do it myself. The one vital piece missing was the correct starter motor. The Blue Spot had a reverse throw starter and I eventually found one in a scrapyard in the Midlands.

Putting the engine back in the car was much more difficult than taking it out as there was only an inch or two to spare and lining up the splines of the drive shaft a nightmare to avoid bending the shaft. In the end it was ready to run and this it did, much to my surprise, very quickly. It ran for about two minutes and then stopped suddenly. One of the valves that I had so carefully ground in had stuck. I hit the top of the valve smartly with a hammer and the engine started straight away and gave no further trouble all the rest of the time I had the car.

Life was looking up and all that I needed to do now was to get the next rung up the training ladder by getting a Registrar's post in General Surgery. Here the omens were not so good as I failed at the first attempt. Professor Smith assured me that all I needed to do was stay in a holding job and I would eventually get a Registrar's post in Aberdeen when 'it was my turn'. I negotiated to stay on in Casualty for a second six months simply to keep me in a paid job.

Muriel and I had resolved that we would be a thoroughly modern family and take Jake, as he'd by now been nicknamed, with us as much as possible. To do this we needed to change our car and traded the

Sport in for a red Saab estate. This was a rather unusual design and although it did not have the same sporty feel it had a lot of room in it.

In the spring two Registrar posts came up but much to my despair I didn't get either. I knew that I must move up soon or I would be in the position of being too old for Surgery. When I failed to get the next one either I began to get annoyed, and suspicious that I was not getting sufficient support. The only alternative was to seek jobs away from Aberdeen and I started to apply for all the jobs advertised in the *British Medical Journal.*

Sadly at this time Muriel's father James died. He was one of the nicest men I have ever met and the last few years saw him an unhappy man. He was retired from a long career as a single handed GP practising from No. 9. In the first War, before studying medicine, he had been a Lead Sergeant in the Horse Artillery. He had kept his Colt 45 revolver, and some ammunition, as well as a captured German Luger automatic pistol which had no firing pin. We handed them in after his death.

He had suffered from stomach ulcers all his life and at some stage had had a Polya radical gastrectomy. This had left him with dreadful side effects including sickness, dumping and diarrhoea, after even the smallest of meals. He survived mainly on a diet of McEwans Export beer. He and I shared many a can well into the night as we talked about all the subjects under the sun.

He became weaker and weaker and was eventually taken into Aberdeen Royal Infirmary. He literally faded away. I was only slightly surprised when 'anorexia' was on his death certificate. I talked to his consultant about it and he was in no doubt about it. I missed him greatly.

The first job I applied for was on a training rotation in Oxford and the second one on a rotation in Bristol. The former appeared the more prestigious as it involved cardiac surgery and working on the professorial unit. I was short-listed for both and found that the Oxford interview was first with Bristol the very next day. I resolved to await the outcome of Oxford before deciding about going to Bristol.

I was offered the Oxford post on the spot and accepted it. Only having done so did I discover that I would be expected to sleep in the intensive care unit with the patients after their cardiac surgery. I had done this with the dialysis patients in Aberdeen and had no desire to do it again at the age of thirty-one. They had not specified this requirement in the advertisement, nor the job description, so I told them that I didn't want the job after all. It turned out to be my lucky day.

I went on to Bristol and had a very difficult and stiff interview the next day. To my surprise I was offered one of the jobs on the Frenchay

– Southmead Senior House Officer Rotational Training Scheme. I was to find out later, and from my own experiences, that this was, and possibly still is, one of the best in the whole country.

Two members of the panel who had given me a particularly hard grilling were both crusty Scotsmen, Colin Davidson and Dougie Milne. Colin told me, afterwards, that most of the panel thought I was too old but he had pushed for me, and Dougie had agreed to take me for my first job. He also advised me not to use Professor Smith as a referee. This devastated me after all the promises he had been making to me in Aberdeen. It taught me a lesson that I passed on to all my trainees in the future which is to ask for 'support for an application' not 'a reference'. This later allows the writer to give a poor or bad one, unknown to the candidate.

I left Aberdeen on 31 July 1968 to start my Surgical Training proper in Bristol. It was a decision that I was later to consider one of the best in my life.

Surgical Training: Bristol, 1968–1971

FRENCHAY HOSPITAL is a very busy General Hospital, with a Major Accident department, Plastic and Thoracic Surgery, and Neurosurgery. I shared the Thoracic job with Paul Preece, later to be Senior Lecturer in Dundee. We only looked after Mr Milne's patients who were down one side of the Nightingale wards with Mr Belsay's down the other. The two did not speak to each other at all, I never discovered why.

We had to act as housemen, as there was no one else to do it, but we were also expected to manage the patients and be in theatre for all the lists. Many of the thoracic operations took a long time and at first I was the 2nd assistant. This meant leaning on a retractor, usually pulling on the ribs, for hours on end and getting shouted at if relaxing at all. The first assistant on our side was the senior registrar Mr Jaysingham, a delightful Indian who replaced Mr Milne when he died, several years later.

The nurses on the wards, and ourselves, cared for all the complicated requirements of the patients post operatively, and thought little of it. There was a strict routine for the timing of removal of the inter-costal drains, and if not removed within 48 hours, they were re-sited by us under local anaesthetic.

If any chest X-rays needed to be done at weekends we had to do them ourselves as the radiographers did not have time. We wet processed them and had them ready for Mr Milne to see at coffee time on Saturdays and Sundays. Mr Milne was, at the time, Chairman of Bristol Rovers Football Club.

In the first month I lived in the Mess while I looked round for a house for us. We sold No. 60 for £5,260 in the days before Aberdeen became an oil town. Muriel came down for a long weekend, with Jake, and we found a new house, not yet completed, in Alveston, near

Thornbury, a few miles north on the A38 (the M5 motorway had not been built). The price of the house was to be £7,500 so that we had to take a mortgage for £3,500 with the Halifax.

Mess life was entirely different to that in Aberdeen and much more reminiscent of Naval Mess life, but in a much more relaxed atmosphere. The food was excellent and many Consultants ate there at lunchtimes. A lot of the medical staff lived in, mostly just when on call but a few permanently if they were single, or their wives were elsewhere.

The heterosexual activity in the mess was intense. There were single doctors sleeping with single nurses, married doctors sleeping with single nurses, married nurses sleeping with single doctors and married doctors, and in one instance a married doctor sleeping with two nurses together. We were served early morning tea by the steward who asked if you wished 'one cup or two today, Doctor?'

We moved into 62 Lime Grove towards the end of September. There were a lot of families on the estate of our age and we made a lot of friends very quickly. On our left, in the end house, No. 63, were the Raymonts, he worked for the BBC; on our right, in No. 61, were the Hargreaves, he worked at Thornbury power-station and was a fanatical gardener.

In the row behind lived the local GP Mike Watts and his wife Jill; John and Sylvena Saul (he worked for the Civil Aviation Association on certifying Concorde); John and Gill Allan (Chief Flight Engineer on Concorde). Along the road were Neil and Linda Evans (a turbine blade designer with Bristol, later Rolls Royce, engines and she was an actress). Opposite us lived Dr John Zorrab, who was Colin Davidson's anaesthetist.

The job was very busy and as well as the routine operations we would get a number of trauma victims with chest injuries. Once we had got the hang of the operations Mr Milne began to let us open and close the chest. I found this was an invaluable technique to have learned.

He was a meticulous operator and he hated to see a single red cell go to waste. I am sure this contributed to his low post-operative complication rate. The main suture materials we used in those days were catgut and silk. Mr Milne, however, used stainless steel wire. Learning to tie those knots was a nightmare.

The Jaguar was too wide to be able to drive it fast and safely down the country lanes. I sold it to Jocelyn Cadbury, the only car I think I have ever sold for a profit. I have always regretted selling it, more especially when he later committed suicide. I bought a Triumph GT6 instead.

I worked at Christmas and was off for New Year. Muriel went up to Aberdeen with Jake, Roger and the cat in time for Christmas leaving me to fend for myself for a week. On New Year's Eve I drove to Aberdeen in the GT6 and I had taken some annual leave into the beginning of January. Muriel's mother was thrilled to have not only Jake but also Alex who was Jean and Hamish's first child, a honeymoon baby, and Christopher, their second child who aged with Jake.

I soon learned how important it is for all surgeons to know how to open the chest quickly when we admitted a man who had been stabbed through the heart; the carving knife was still sticking out of his chest and was going up and down with each heartbeat. Mr Milne simply put a strong catgut purse string stitch round the blade deeply through the heart muscle and then told me to pull the knife out quickly.

A man impaled himself on some railings in the centre of Bristol and the fire brigade had had to cut him free. Mr Milne got to Frenchay before the patient and again we simply pulled the steel rod out.

On 1 February 1969 I started the second job on the rotation, six months General Surgery at Southmead Hospital with Michael Wilson, a General Surgeon with an interest in vascular surgery. It is on the north side of Bristol near where Concorde was under construction. Roger Eltringham, a New Zealander, a Senior Lecturer, was the other Consultant.

Like many of the surgeons in Bristol Mr Wilson had a large private practice and would operate down at the Convent Nursing Home at least twice a week. One day he had a hemi-thyroidectomy for the first case on the list at Southmead which I was to start while he did a 'small' case at the Convent. I completed my first thyroid operation before he arrived. The patient was none the worse I'm pleased to say.

I was helping Mr Wilson in the Convent one day. When the operation was finished and we were ready to stitch up the count did not tally, with three small swabs missing. After several counts, we still could not find them and had searched the patient's abdomen thoroughly several times. A young Novice then admitted that she had thrown the three skin preparation swabs into the bin. As penance she was made to search the rubbish until she found them.

There were peripheral clinics in Wells, Somerset, and Cleveden, on alternate fortnights. These involved travelling down by car, on a Wednesday, in time for lunch, which in Wells was at the house of the local GP who also gave the anaesthetics in the afternoon. The lunch was accompanied by a bottle of wine. Ether was used for the anaesthetic so that no diathermy was allowed. The problem was being fit and safe to drive home after all the alcohol and ether.

There was a Paediatric unit at Southmead and for the first time I was involved in seeing children in the acute situation other than trauma. I was frequently summoned to remove an appendix when it was obvious that the child did not have appendicitis: usually constipation, but sometimes something much worse like Crohn's disease or lymphoma.

One of the worst differences of opinions was over the management of neo-natal pyloric stenosis. It is common practice to operate on these immediately the diagnosis is made and it is a small procedure with few complications. Here they were put on Ephedrene in the belief that this would cause relaxation of the sphincter. This treatment rarely, if ever, worked but it did make it very soggy making the operation much more difficult and hazardous.

One of the worst aspects of the job was a Varicose Vein Clinic every Friday afternoon. It was always the task of the poor SHO to do. One lady with a tiny superficial vein on her thigh was outraged at my suggestion that, in order for her to wear her bikini, she should use body make up. Hers was, I believe, the first official complaint against me by a patient.

Mr Wilson's hobby was dinghy sailing and the incumbent SHO was expected to crew for him. I pre-empted the request by buying my own GP14 for £100. *Alouette* is an old wooden boat, No. 1138. She is now on the Forth being sailed by my son and his friend, after two rebuilds.

There was great excitement in the hospital when we learned that the British Concorde was to take to the air for the first time around lunchtime on 9 April 1970. I had a list to do that afternoon and reluctantly went up to start. We had a radio on in the scrub room and when the news came that they were about to take off we all downed tools and rushed to the end window overlooking the runway. Only when we turned round did we realise that the only people still in the theatres were the two unconscious patients on the anaesthetic ventilators.

In the midst of all this activity I was trying to study for the Fellowship and again realised that my practical skills and knowledge far outweighed the theoretical knowledge I would need to pass the exam. I bought a new 'Bailey and Love' and started a card index for each topic in the book. I could see that one of my greatest limiting factors was going to be Orthopaedics which is an amazingly large subject.

We were within easy driving distance of a lot of our old friends and went to visit them whenever my rota allowed. Graham and Wendy Reid now lived at Larkhill, the Royal Artillery Base, where he was the Adjutant. Although I had held his Medical Records in my office in the Far East I had had no cause to need to see them and was shocked to hear that he had had Hodgkin's Disease. He had just had a relapse and gone to Millbank Military Hospital and then Greenwich for treatment.

Most of our neighbours went camping for their summer holidays. We bought a large blue frame tent with two bedrooms and a large living space, and an open fronted frame cooking tent with cooker, larder etc. We put all this up in the garden but to get a real feel for this sort of camping we went to Symonds Yat, just over the border into Wales, to try it all out. We had no sooner put the tent up than it started to rain and by the following morning the campsite was a sea of mud. We packed quickly and returned home, resolving only to camp in warmer climates.

For this we chose Brittany. We packed the camping gear in the boat and drove down to Concarneau. We were not certain what the weather would be like or how Jake would take to camping so Muriel had arranged for her mother and Aunt Alice to fly down to Quimper where they stayed in a hotel. This arrangement worked well and we were able to have baths in their room and we sometimes left Jake overnight so that we were not tied.

The next part of the rotation was Urology at Ham Green, an old fever hospital, to the south-west of Bristol. I worked for Roger Fenneley and Humphrey White, a Senior Lecturer in Transplantation. The Urology was very specialised here and related to working up the patients, with the Nephrologist, Campbell McKenzie, for consideration for transplanting which was still in its infancy in those days.

It was apparent that the crucial part of the procedure was to do a good tunnelled implantation to prevent leakage or reflux to damage the new kidney. Once mastered the operation is a simple one in the pelvis and after having done a few I found them rather boring although obviously life saving for the patients. Rejection was the biggest complication.

Kidneys for the transplants were, as now, in short supply and came to Ham Green in taxis with no special boxes but simply in kidney dishes in ice. One day we were waiting in theatre with the patient ready to have the kidney implanted but it didn't arrive. Frantically we phoned the taxi firm who discovered that the driver had picked up a passenger on his way across and forgotten about the kidney. Luckily the kidney was still there, we implanted it and the patient was none the worse.

The social life at Ham Green was, if anything, wilder than at either of the other two hospitals. A nurse fancied one of our housemen; she was about 5 feet tall, and he about 6ft 2ins. She made a pass at him and they disappeared upstairs to his room. A short time later there was a loud scream. The nurse was down to her bra and pants, and our colleague to his pants, but it was he who was screaming and was cowering on top of his bed-head shouting for us to get her away. We were all very bemused indeed.

I returned to Southmead in November. I was working with the senior Urologist Norman Slade, and Michael Roberts. Both were involved in the development of the optical instruments that were to revolutionise Urology. In those days the equipment was very primitive with hard lenses, mirrors and light bulbs at the end of the instrument. Although only a 12 volt system, it was easy to get small burns on the nose from short circuits.

They were also at the forefront of transurethral resection of the prostate with variants of this equipment. I could see the value of this in avoiding a scar but it took a long time to remove a large prostate.

Mr Slade did these new TURs, as they were called, privately for 100 guineas (£105). The Chairman of Wills Tobacco Company was referred to him and it was arranged for him to have it done in the Private Hospital on Saturday morning. We, the SHOs, were asked to assist and we got paid £10. I arrived this Saturday to learn that the Chairman had taken himself up to London where he paid 1000 guineas for the same operation.

The sexual activities that I came across continued to have me in awe. One of our housemen had two partners. One was a medical student with whom he shared a flat. The other was a married radiographer who shared his bed at the hospital when he and/or she was on duty. At one fateful party in the Mess the radiographer found him *in flagrante delicto* with the medical student and there was an unholy public row.

As soon as we had arrived in Bristol Muriel and I had told Mike Watts that we wanted to adopt a girl as soon as possible so that there would only be a couple of years between the children. He got us accepted on to the local council adoption scheme but were advised that there was starting to be a shortage of children offered for adoption.

Jake, who had had a squint since birth, had been wearing a patch over his good eye to try to improve the other but without success. He went into the Bristol eye hospital at the age of two and a half to have it straightened. The paediatricians were starting to not wear white coats and the nurse's uniform. I thought that this was yet another detrimental step in the NHS and disagreed that children were afraid of white coats and uniforms. I asked Jake what he thought about the idea of no uniforms. His reply showed how much children take after their parents as he said, 'How would I know who the bloody doctor was?'

I returned to Frenchay Hospital on 1 February 1970. I shared this rota with Pete Curtis with whom I got on very well. I worked, at last for

Colin Davidson and Roger Celestin (of Celestin Tube fame). They like Dougie Milne and Belsay did not speak to each other although they shared wards. I asked Colin, many years later, why they had fallen out and he could not remember; neither could Roger Celestin. They were completely different characters, and personalities, and treated almost everything surgical differently. God help you if you forgot whose patient you were treating.

Colin, to me, was a dour Scotsman very like my father in many ways. Any telling off was quickly forgotten, as long as not repeated. He let me do a lot as an SHO and was really cross with me when he went on holiday once and I did all the thyroids on his waiting list while he was away. I had not realised that was his favourite operation.

Celestin, on the other hand, was a completely different kettle of fish. He let you do no operations, except those out of hours, and wrote all the discharge letters in a way that if all had gone well for the patient he would take the credit and if there was a complication he pointed the finger at the junior concerned.

It was time for me, at the age of 33, to get my Fellowship and I had my first attempt in March 1970. I knew it was a forlorn hope but wanted to get a feel for the exam. I had been correct and failed but not badly enough to be deferred for a year. The next exam was in June and I began to work harder now I had sampled it.

A Registrar's post came vacant later that month and I applied in spite of my exam failure and I got it with much pushing from Colin again who afterwards said I had 'better get the exam now'. I could only work hard at it and hope.

It was spring and I longed for an open sports car so I was extravagant and replaced the GT6 with a new, flame red TR6. It had virtually the same engine as the GT but with two seats and a soft top. It went even faster and would easily overtake MGBs on slip roads.

The local adoption group had found us a baby girl. We collected Fiona Alice when she was a week old. Jake was thrilled and did not go through a jealousy phase. Jake's adoption had gone very smoothly but little did we know the severe emotional trauma that we were later to experience with Fiona's.

I shared the Registrar rotation with two delightful colleagues, Frank MacGinn and John Cochrane. There were nine month slots with Colin Davidson and Roger Celestin and nine months at Cossham, a satellite hospital one and a half miles away, looking after everyone there, including Mr Herbie Bourns from the BRI.

As is usual in life the new boy gets the short straw, and that was the

Cossham job. In my case this was worse than for the other two as they both lived on that side of Frenchay while I lived to the north. It was virtually impossible to give proper cover on take nights without living in. This was two nights a week but 1 in 3 for weekends.

Just after I was appointed there was a party, after work, for the person that I was replacing, I cannot remember his name. Towards the end of the party a stunning, tall, blond 3rd year nurse in uniform, whom I didn't recognise, came in to wish him goodbye. Her name was Jennie and then I remembered her two years previously as a very young, schoolgirlish, first year nurse. Most people decided to go on and have a meal. Jennie said that she would like to but would have to go home and change.

I offered to drive her home and wait for her to get changed. We had a most enjoyable evening. Jennie and I got on well but did not think any further than a friendship developing especially as one of the wags at the party had made the usual male remark: 'You've got no chance there, Ron – she's a very fussy lady.' Charming, I thought.

He was entirely wrong, and that chance meeting led to a relationship that lasted several years, off and on, two job changes and moves on my part, and a disastrous marriage for her. She had no car so I bought her a 'banger', an Austin A30, and even that survived for some time. She was a lovely girl and did not deserve the bad luck which seemed to dog her, culminating in her mother, whom she adored, being seriously ill.

The job at Cossham was enjoyable and busy. Mr Bourns was almost retiring and doing less and less. He was of the old school of surgeons who were 'cutters' and used fewer of the modern ideas that Colin taught. One particular operation he showed me to do using the original Kocher's Cholecystectomy clamps, one for the artery and one for the bile duct and then remove the gall bladder. It took him ten minutes altogether.

I spent much of my spare time studying for the Fellowship which was possible at home as Fiona and Jake went to bed soon after I got there. After supper I would spend a couple of hours studying and felt that I was beginning to have a better theoretical grip. I tried the exam again in Edinburgh in June but failed at the clinical stage having this time passed the theory. I realised that I would have to make a superhuman effort to get it next time, in October, and set about negotiating to go on a refresher course before it.

We had had Fiona a few months by now and were shattered to be told that her natural mother was considering revoking her decision to have her adopted. The mother has this right but it is rarely taken. We would have no real alternative but to comply as the law would support her claim. We were left in a state of shock and being able to do nothing except continue to love and care for Fiona, and hope for the best.

The health authorities did not give study leave for courses and did not pay fees. I took a holiday at the end of six months at Cossham and went up to London for the three week Middlesex Hospital course. The most important point of this course from my point of view was the continual viva questioning by Consultants. This gave me a lot more confidence in responding to questions and when I went up to Edinburgh again on 15 October was certain that this would be my best chance yet.

I passed the written, and the vivas, and had to go back up on 3 November 1970 for the clinicals. In the meantime I sat the writtens in London for the English College. As a Scotsman, and a Scottish graduate, I did not really want an English Fellowship but in Bristol it was deemed impossible to get a Senior Registrar post without it.

I felt very confident during the exam until towards the end when Mr Soutar asked me some very obscure questions. Awaiting the results I became full of trepidation that I had failed yet again and was surprised to be told I had passed. I asked Mr Soutar about the strange questions and he laughed saying that as I had been working in England he wanted to be sure that I had not been learning too many obscure facts rather than the fundamentals.

I was booked on the night sleeper back to London which did not leave till 11 p.m. After phoning Muriel to tell her the good news, I went to a steak bar in Queen Street to have a beer and a meal. There I met three female law students who, when they discovered I had just passed the Fellowship and I was on my own, insisted that I bought a bottle of champagne to celebrate and they would help me drink it. I said that was fine but in return they would have to guarantee to put me on the sleeper. The girls kept their word and I regret never being able to thank them.

I also got to the clinicals in the exam in London and did all right until I met Mr Smydie, from Leeds, who took me on the short cases and I failed on his marking. Poor Pete Curtis also failed on this occasion, for the umpteenth time. The following week as Colin, Pete and I were leaving Cossham after an outpatient clinic, and Colin was congratulating me on my success, and commiserating with Pete, Colin shook us both rigid by alluding to Pete's appetite for the ladies interfering with his studies.

Fiona was approaching six months and we were finally informed that her mother had decided that she wanted her back. We replied that we would not give Fiona back willingly and without a fight. We were again told that we could take it to court for a decision but that it was unlikely that we would win. I let it be known through Mike Watts, the GP, who was the go-between us and the local authority, that we would only return Fiona on a 1 to 1 exchange basis. We would exchange Fiona for another, new, baby there and then.

We were told that they could not accept such terms. 'We'll see you in Court then,' was our reply. After much negotiating they agreed, with bad grace, and we had the traumatic experience of taking Fiona back and returning home with a new one week old girl whom we also called Fiona but changed the spelling of her second name from Alice to Alys for individuality.

It was Jake who was the most traumatised by this and demonstrated it by immediately asking, at the age of three, when HE would have to go back. Jake did not get over this incident for a long time and often would ask that dreadful question. Nothing we could say would convince him that it wasn't going to happen to him ever.

We had further distressing news about this time in that Graham had a further relapse of his Hodgkin's Disease and died. Wendy and he had only been married for a few years and although she had come to realise that he was losing the battle was none the less distressed.

Roger, the springer, had also died at a great age. In the light of all the other changes in the family we thought that we needed to replace him immediately. We thought that a change of breed was needed and went in search of an Old English sheepdog. We found one which we named Garth after the cartoon character. He was as big as Roger when we got him at three months and grew rapidly. Although large, he was surprisingly gentle with the children and we never felt that he was any danger to them and he rapidly became very protective of them.

The family went to Aberdeen as usual for Christmas. I joined them for New Year. Having got over the shock of meeting a new, younger Fiona, the family fell for her. I have always hoped that the first Fiona had a good life with her natural mother and that it was the right decision on the mother's part to want her back.

In the New Year I returned to Frenchay to work with Colin. Life was becoming a bit more normal as I was able to stay at home when I was on call and Frenchay was not on take. Mr Bourns retired and a new appointment made who was also going to work at Frenchay. We took great interest in all the candidates who came to look over the job. We were least impressed by one who came down from London in his Rolls Royce and looked down his nose at us from the provinces. Luckily his Rolls Royce was too wide for the narrow bridge to Cossham.

Roy May was appointed and he obviously did not know about the rift between Colin and Roger Celestin but quickly found out who was his friend. I also looked after his patients. We admitted a patient who had a ruptured kidney. Roy was on duty and I called him in. I was surprised when in theatre he admitted that he had never done any Urology. He came from St James, Balham, a mainly gastroenterological unit, and I nervously removed the kidney with him assisting me.

Wendy, after Graham's death, came down to stay with us and we decided to hold a party that weekend. We invited all my colleagues and their wives. John Cochrane was separated and in the middle of a messy divorce at the time. At the end of the evening, about 2 a.m., we found them both sitting on the stairs as we were clearing up. It turned out that they had got on like a house on fire and John, not realising she was staying with us, was waiting for her to leave before he did.

We learned, with a bit of a chuckle, that he had asked her back the following weekend and that she had stayed with him. She is 5ft nothing and he is 6ft 4ins. We were very happy for both of them as they both needed this sort of happiness. They married and now live in Edinburgh where John was a hand surgeon until his recent retiral.

I had missed the Navy/Marine camaraderie and approached the Bristol Marine Reserve Unit to see if they wanted a Commando trained doctor. They did and wondered why I had waited the five years to become involved. No one, of course, had told me that you can be on the Emergency List and the RNR. I joined List 5 in which one is expected to do so many 'drill nights' and two weeks continuous training a year, all of which earns pay.

We were asked by some of the neighbours if we would like to join some of them camping in northern Mediterranean Spain at Tamarui. Having spent all that money on the camping gear we decided to give it a go especially as they all assured us that the weather was both hot and dry all the time. It was only a short walk down to the village which in those days was still a small fishing village with but one small hotel and a few restaurants and bars. There was a lovely beach and a sheltered cove where I noticed there was a small sailing club.

We thoroughly enjoyed ourselves and I took the opportunity to re-grow my beard during this three week holiday. Fiona, although so young, was no problem. At night, after feeding the children and getting them ready for bed, one couple would stay and babysit whilst the rest went out for a meal. The couple remaining were liberally supplied with alcohol so there was no real hardship to do this every fourth night.

We decided to return across the base of the Pyrenees on the French side. From Gerona we climbed up into Andorra which was shrouded in thick cloud. Jake asked, 'When will we reach the moon?' The weather really remained the same as we drove to Pau, where we stayed the night and then back into Spain before staying the last night in San Sebastián. We ate a Spanish tortilla for our supper and both got severe food poisoning such that it took all our will power to drive the short distance along the coast to Bilbao and the ferry home.

Colin was not at all impressed with my beard and viewed it with suspicion as far as wound infections were concerned. I kept a very careful note of all the wounds in the next few months and next time he mentioned it was able to report that my record was better than his own. There were over a hundred hernias on his waiting list awaiting repair. I put together a little project to do four hernias twice a week using the same beds. The patients had clips in the wounds instead of stitches and these were taken out after only 48 hours when they were sent home. We cleared the waiting list in three months and there were no serious problems with the wounds.

I spent my two weeks' continuous training with the Royal Naval Reserve on Salisbury Plain as medical cover for the Marines who came from all over the country. It was customary for there to be a farewell party on the Friday night before they all went home. As no party is much fun without female company, I approached the matrons of the local hospitals. They agreed to allow me to put up a notice on their notice boards as long as I provided transport to and from the camp. Bets were placed that I would fail and as the party got under way there was no sign of the bus or girls. Half an hour late I arrived with the bus almost full of nurses to be greeted with much cheering.

In view of my extensive clinical experience at SHO level, I did not wish to stay in the Registrar post for more than 18 months if I was to make up any time in my career pathway. Colin did not think I would get a Senior Registrar job in the South West and advised me to go and do a Research job. This was something that I had not considered but Colin had a lot of contacts and suggested that I approach Professor Pat Forrest who had only recently moved from Cardiff to replace Sir John Bruce in Edinburgh.

A job was advertised in the late autumn which I applied for. I was called for an interview, shaved off my beard, again, in order to enhance my chances, and was appointed with the objective of doing an MD in some aspects of breast cancer research.

I left Bristol in late November and started in the Royal Infirmary immediately. There were several farewell parties, not least of all the one in the Hospital where I was surprised and delighted when all the staff clubbed together and presented me with a silver beer tankard. We put the house on the market and then started to move our bits and pieces back up to No. 9 in Aberdeen. This somewhat precipitous move to Edinburgh also turned out to be one of the most important of my career and I shall always be indebted to Colin, not only for his surgical training, but for paving the way with Professor Forrest.

CHAPTER THIRTEEN

Research: Edinburgh, 1971–1973

I STARTED in the Professorial Unit in Edinburgh Royal Infirmary on 1 December 1971. I had expected to be doing research but my appointment letter was for a straight Surgical Registrar post. The clinical work was no different from all my other jobs but here you had to justify every decision and I could see that I was going to have to sharpen my wits to survive in this academic environment.

There was also a distinct 'atmosphere' between the new Professor and the remaining 'Edinburgh' staff of the unit. Another 'atmosphere' existed between the Surgical Unit and the non-academic surgical units, and the rest of the hospital. Within the Unit there was distress that the Chair had not gone to one of the two Senior Lecturers, either Tom Hamilton or Ian McLeod, and that the metabolic and trauma research of the department, under Sir John Bruce with Bill Gill and Howard Champion, would close and be replaced by breast cancer research.

Bob Buchan, an Aberdeen graduate, was one of the lecturers and John Chamberlain, the Senior Registrar on the Vascular Unit, who, soon after we met, went to a Consultant post in Newcastle-upon-Tyne. Colin Currie (Colin Douglas) had just published his semi-factual novel *The Houseman's Tale*, based round an outbreak of hepatitis in the Infirmary. When they made the book into a film they recreated the atmosphere exactly.

One of the sillier confrontational points between the Unit and the rest was the wearing of the collar of the white coat 'up' by the Unit and in the normal 'down' position by the rest. The foremost exponent of this was Ian McLeod, nicknamed 'stiff lips' because of the rarity of his smile. In fact he is a very nice person.

There were two main options for after-work relaxation. The first was a corner pub immediately opposite the hospital which was then called 'The Mortar' but is now known as 'The Doctor', since *The Houseman's Tale* was made into a film. The second was just a few hundred yards

down the road at the University Club. It was here that I first met Sir
John Bruce – with his trouser flies undone showing blue and white
striped boxer shorts beneath.

Tom Hamilton moved to a job in Perth, Western Australia, and Bill
Gill and Howard Champion to a Trauma Centre in Maryland, USA.
Once they had settled in they offered me a post as Associate Professor
but I did not feel inclined to spend the rest of my life in Trauma or
America.

I found myself on duty over Christmas and only got off in time to
drive up to Aberdeen leaving at 6 a.m. on New Year's morning. The
journey in the TR6 was very quick and I only saw two other vehicles
in the whole 150 miles. The family had moved up to Aberdeen while
we found a new house in Edinburgh. The prices in 1971 were still
reasonable and we had put in a bid for a house in Morningside, one of
the posh parts of Edinburgh.

I only had a couple of days leave, being the new boy, and on return
to the Unit I was asked by APMF, as we called Professor Forrest, if I
was coming to the SRS. The Surgical Research Society was a totally new
experience for me and the aggressive questioning of the speakers was the
same as occurred back in the Unit except in front of an audience of
several hundred. I learned that anyone expecting to make it in Surgery
had to give a paper here. I shuddered at the thought.

We got occupancy of 66 Cluny Gardens in the middle of January
1972. It was a typical Edinburgh stone built semi-detached house that
backed onto the Blackford Hill Park. The main disadvantage was that
it lay on a main road and the drive opened straight onto it making it
difficult to reverse a car in or out, and dangerous for the children. We
paid £11,000 for the property. It was handy for Morningside junior
school, which Jake would be going to in September, and for the park
to exercise Garth.

Muriel found a stable nearby and moved the, by now, two horses
into it. It was part of a farm and they had some geese. The gander was
a real nuisance and would attack almost anyone and try to bite their
ankles. The best safeguard was a broom to keep it at a distance and it
was not long before Jake learned this technique; at this stage I almost
became sorry for the goose.

There was at that time a Royal Naval Reserve Unit in Leith, HMS
Claverhouse, to which I transferred. Their main interest was in mine-
sweeping and there was no Marine Unit, the nearest being in Dundee.
I did as many drills as I felt would satisfy the rules for my annual bounty
payment and unlike the previous social life in Bristol found them a

pretty snobbish lot. The only really cheerful face, albeit mainly covered by a black beard, was Colin Currie. He went on to do a long attachment to the Royal Navy between NHS jobs, serving on a frigate during one of the Iceland Cod Wars, and wrote his second book *Wellies for the Queen* based on those experiences.

When March arrived and there was still no sign of me getting to start any research I asked to see the Professor. My interview with him was about 8 a.m. He asked if I was enjoying the Unit and then I explained that I had come to his Unit to do research, not more clinical work. 'Do you really want to do Surgery?' he asked.

'Yes Sir,' I replied.

'In that case you had better start reading about the hormone Prolactin for the next three months and then you can start your research. In the meantime Bob Buchan is going to have to take three months sick leave and I want you to take over his clinical duties.'

My mind, working quicker than normal at this time of day, reminded me that Bob was a Lecturer with Senior Registrar status. 'That's fine, Sir,' I said, 'but I would like to act up to his clinical grading if I'm deemed capable of doing the job.'

'Right,' replied the Professor, 'but will you please stop calling me "Sir".'

'What should I call you then?' I asked politely.

'Professor when we meet for the first time in the Unit in the morning and Pat socially,' he replied. That, I thought, should present no problems, and it didn't until he was knighted.

Bob Buchan's job posed no real problem for me although it caused problems when I had to venture off the Unit to see patients in other parts and Units of the hospital as I was seen as Professor Forrest's boy and they were not used to major clinical decisions being taken by a complete stranger.

Two cases spring to mind. The first was an obstetric one in a lady with appendicitis due to deliver in only two weeks time. My opposite number in Obstetrics was not at all keen to let me go ahead and operate and got his Consultant to come in. He was a very nice man, a good obstetrician, and agreed with me. She went on to have a normal delivery two weeks later.

The second case related to a severe haemorrhage following a small bowel biopsy taken by a small device called a Crosby Capsule that the patient swallows and a tiny knife, activated by applying a vacuum, removes a sample of the lining. There is a possibility of a rather deep cut occurring that may lead to haemorrhage. This, statistically, happens about once in every 200 cases.

The juniors again disagreed with my diagnosis, and sent for their Consultant. He was one of the characters portrayed in *The Houseman's Tale* and although I had never met him before immediately recognised him from the book: 'his patients never bled like this.' I enquired, as politely as possible, how many he had done. The answer '198' surprised even me.

Professor Forrest had established a dedicated breast clinic as soon as he arrived in Edinburgh and, in this, he was supported by Maureen Roberts, who had come up from Cardiff and was now leading his new research team. Much of the research interest was in female steroid hormones and their possible roles in breast cancer. Oestrogen receptors were in their early days of clinical interest and these were analysed in the laboratories across the road, in the University, by Bill Miller.

New drugs were also undergoing clinical trial in the Unit and we had ICI 46474, later to be called Tamoxifen. We were doing a double blind trial with it against Stilboestrol. The two identical containers had 'T' and 'S' stamped on the bottom so it was not difficult to tell who was on which drug. When it came to pill compliance the Tamoxifen bottles were empty since it is free of side effects in the post-menopausal woman. The Stilboestrol bottles would come back more than half full as they made the women universally sick.

Tamoxifen has been referred to as an oestrogen blocking drug and everyone wanted to measure the receptors in the belief that this would pick out the patients who would respond to it. In reality it doesn't work quite like that and the main clinical value of the receptor measurement was for prognosis of the disease. The same information can be gained from careful histological examination of the tumour at much less expense and more quickly.

I spent as much time as I could during this time reading about Prolactin. There had been very little work done on this hormone until recently when it had been discovered that rodent mammary tumours could be manipulated in their growth behaviour, or even prevented, by changing its level. There was great excitement among the animal physiologists at this finding.

I am not an anti-vivisectionist, as I believe that it is not possible safely to go from the test-tube to the human in one move, but firmly believe that there are fundamental differences between rodents (and monkeys even) and humans, not least of all the presence (or absence) of a long tail.

Measurement of the hormone levels, in the 1970s, largely relied on radio-immunoassay techniques. The limiting factor was the availability of some of the pure hormone to inject into a rabbit that then produced antibodies to the foreign species hormone. There had been no source of the human pituitary glands from which it is secreted, and can be extracted, until a very small supply of nearly pure Prolactin antibody arrived from America at the Tenovus Institute in Cardiff.

The Prolactin (HPr) assay itself was going to be done in Cardiff so I was going to spend a lot of time commuting. The children were getting bigger and I needed more room in my car so I changed my TR6 for a new, mustard-coloured Triumph Stag. I would leave Edinburgh about 6 a.m. and arrive in Cardiff in time to meet my colleagues from the laboratory for lunch in the local hospital pub.

I was given the privilege of a free run of thought, required for an MD thesis, as to how to establish if there was any link between blood levels of Prolactin and human breast cancer. There was no shortage of patients willing to participate in almost anything that might help in breast cancer research.

The only British expert in Prolactin chose this moment to leave and go to Canada as his employer did not see the value of his current direction of research into the function(s) of Prolactin. Since it is one of the most primitive hormones, and its effects were little understood, this seemed to be a particularly short-sighted decision on their part.

I first measured the resting circulation level in several dozen people of both sexes, of all ages, and with and without breast disease (benign and malignant). I, personally, was not really surprised to find that everyone, including us males, had very similar, low levels. This contrasted to the high levels seen in rats with induced breast tumours.

This piece of work, upsetting the rodent workers as it did, was my first presentation paper at the Endocrine Section of the Royal Society of Medicine. This was quite frightening enough on its own but I had not realised that the audience was almost entirely made up of eminent Medical Endocrinologists.

I noticed that if the patient, or volunteer, was apprehensive or downright frightened their levels rose almost instantly to enormous levels. I asked myself what was the physiological purpose of this but had to get back to investigating its role in breast cancer. I found that, like most hormones, there was a diurnal rhythm of secretion in all groups of patients and normals, by persuading medical students to stay cooped up in a laboratory for twenty-four hours. It cost me a lot in beer money.

Exoginous oestrogens produced a marked rise in the plasma level but there appeared to be no correlation between this and a response to the therapy: very negative and disappointing research. The phenothyazine drugs, used in depression, were known to elevate Prolactin in animals and long term female mental patients have an increased incidence of breast cancer. I measured as many of those patients as I could find, and persuade to agree, in the Royal Edinburgh Hospital, including in the locked ward where getting agreement from the patient to take a blood sample could be hazardous. The levels of Prolactin were all raised and there was no difference in the small number of depressives with breast cancer on phenothyazine; nor did I find any cases of male breast cancer.

The Saab estate was becoming too small, with the two children, so we had traded it in for a sand-coloured second-hand Volvo estate. We felt that the drive from Edinburgh to Portsmouth and then down to Spain was really too far with two young children so we opted to go back to Denmark. Our friends lent us their beach house in Rovieg, in the north of Zealand.

On returning to work I next turned my attention to dynamic studies of Prolactin using stimulation and ablation techniques. I looked at the immediate effects with injecting phenothyazines into normal volunteers, and those with all types of breast disease. There was no noticeable between the groups in the quick rise of levels.

In September I arranged my two weeks annual training at ITCRM Lympstone as a relief doctor. I drove down in the Stag and settled back into Marine life, at Lympstone, with ease and found that a lot of the officers I had served with were actually now on the staff. I was pleased to see Dickie Grant, who had let me go ahead with the Commando Course and was currently CO. It turned out he was leaving the Marines to set up a climbing school in Scotland.

The first Friday I was there was to be his Dining Out to which he immediately invited me. I did not have my mess kit, nor a dinner suit, with me but he organised for a collection of clothes. The jacket and the trousers did not come from the same suit and I only had an ordinary white shirt and bow tie. I looked fairly scruffy. To my extreme embarrassment I found myself sat on his right hand side, on the very corner of the top table where I had been squeezed in, with his wife on the other side. Needless to say this caused quite a stir among the Regulars, most of whom didn't know who I was from Adam.

On the second Friday there was a large parade to which I was invited to swell the ranks of the Naval contingent. This consisted of about eight of us and being the Senior Service were spread thinly in front of the three sides of the parade. I had a wasp hovering about the end of my nose for much of the parade but remained calm. It was at the end that the Navy excelled itself by responding to the order to dismiss by turning right, saluting and marching off smartly in the direction of the Mess for a beer. We had all forgotten that the Marines do this in two stages and the first is just the Senior Officer handing the control of the parade to the parade commander who then dismisses the officers.

The initial negative findings meant I needed to expand my research if I was to have enough to get my MD. APMF was well known for his method of pituitary ablation for advanced, mainly bony, breast cancer using Yttrium 90 inserted into the gland, stereotactically, through the nose. This destroys the gland, and Prolactin as a result should disappear from the circulation. The opposite effect on Prolactin production is achieved by pituitary stalk section, favoured in America, and also used in the same group of patients. This results in uncontrolled Prolactin secretion. There was no correlation between the patient's response to either therapy and the resultant Prolactin level.

It was about this time in my research when we got wind of how the pituitaries for the extraction of the Prolactin had actually been obtained in America. The answer was not a very palatable or pleasant one, and the supply abruptly ceased. We were only handling the antibody in extremely careful laboratory conditions as the possibility of transmission of CJD was a known risk in those days. It is sad to think that in the excitement of being able to give human growth hormone (HGH), extracted from the same pituitaries, to under-grown children this risk was initially either ignored or forgotten. I lost a surgical colleague from CJD in his thirties following therapy with HGH given about the time I was doing this research.

I was by now tired of negative research although it was important to have ruled out circulating Prolactin levels as a major influence in human breast cancer. I asked Professor Forrest if I could try to develop a test that would allow him to assess the completeness of his Yttrium 90 ablations.

An insulin induced hypoglycaemia stimulates Prolactin secretion. Initially I used an injection of insulin but this produced such unpredictable effects that I replaced it with a slow infusion with careful monitoring of the glucose level as it fell. The patients underwent the test before the implant and again after it.

I would not exactly call my findings a discovery, but like all good discoveries it is the unexpected that is so exciting. Firstly I found that some ladies with very advanced disease had spontaneously stopped producing Prolactin and were often so unwell that they were not fit enough for the operation, and died soon after. This I believe is due to infiltration of the Pituitary with tumour cells, which is demonstrable at Post Mortem, and I believe indicates who is terminally ill with the disease. It also explains how some women who seem to be coping with their breast cancer suddenly die from Pituitary failure. The second observation was that as the blood glucose fell Prolactin was stimulated before growth hormone. Why should Prolactin be more sensitive?

In June 1973 the first international conference on Human Prolactin was held in Brussels. I arrived at the conference hotel in the late afternoon. Glancing through the programme I saw to my horror that I appeared to be giving a paper the following morning.

APMF had taught us to carry our slides with us, so I sat in the main square of Brussels writing my paper assisted by several bottles of Stella Artois. I had not drunk this before and did not realise just how strong it is. I got back to the hotel to be asked by the doorman if I would like a 'hot water bottle'. Not being cold I said no thanks and not till the next morning did I realise what was meant by his suggestion.

The rodent workers were not impressed by my negative findings in the human and remained convinced of the connection, so much so that they proposed that we set up a project where we took 20,000 pubertal girls and sterilised half of them to demonstrate that they would not get breast cancer in later life. I, having delivered my paper, shot to my feet and suggested that it might be difficult to persuade 10,000 girls and their mothers to volunteer for this experiment.

Muriel and I again decided to go with the group to Tamarui and I decided to take the boat down as we were going for a full three weeks and the tentage travelled inside the boat, giving more room in the car. I was able to go out sailing every day, as long as the wind was not too strong, usually on my own which I really loved, but occasionally with Jake in a lifejacket that was twice his size.

It was on this visit that I became aware that there was a certain amount of wife swapping going on among the group that, on this occasion, was at least five or six couples. We did not participate in this activity but there started to be nights where the couple remaining to baby-sit were not necessarily married and there were 'skinny dipping' expeditions to the beach at midnight.

After we had returned from the holiday we were a little taken aback when two of the families, each with two or three children, swapped fathers. This was simply achieved by the men moving across the road, diagonally, from one house to the other. The whole lot then continued their lives as if nothing had happened.

After nearly eighteen months of research work I had enough to write a thesis. The question as to what Prolactin actually does in the human

I was not able to pursue as I was funded for cancer research only. It was some years before it was realised that Prolactin is the explanation of the anomaly whereby both sodium and potassium are preserved in stress and trauma. A balance is usually struck between positive ions, one rising when the other falls.

I wondered if Prolactin had anything to do with jet lag, it being such a basic hormone. In this I was to be shown wrong as it turns out to be Melatonin. I tried, unsuccessfully, to persuade British Airways to let me sample blood from their air hostesses on a round the world flight. Some you win and some you lose!

I now needed to get back into clinical surgery at Senior Registrar grade. Due to the antipathy between the Unit and the rest of the surgeons in Edinburgh it was unlikely that I would get one there. (I also hadn't gone to Fettes, sung in the Festival choir, nor supported Hearts or Hibs.) A Lecturer in Surgery post was advertised in Nottingham, which was then a new Medical School and their first students were just about to enter the clinical phase of their training. Tom Balfour, who had been in Edinburgh at the Western Infirmary for a short time after I arrived, had gone there as the first lecturer.

APMF supported my decision to apply and I was shortlisted. The day before the interviews I was invited to come and look round the Department that specialised in gastrointestinal research. Another part of the Department, at the City Hospital across town, specialised in renal transplantation and breast cancer.

Professor Jack Hardcastle, from the London Hospital, was the head of Department with Jim Bourke as his Senior Lecturer and Professor Roger Blamey at the City Hospital. I had one of the most exhausting and nerve-racking afternoons I had ever spent. At the end Jim Bourke took me to a pub for a beer(s) and a snack before I spent the night in the residence at the City Hospital.

The next morning the interview was at the University and I approached it with severe trepidation in the light of the grilling I had gone through the previous day. When it was my turn for interview I was dismayed when I was asked few questions and most of those were social ones. About the only serious one that I can remember was the old chestnut as to whether, at the age of now thirty-seven, I really wanted to go on in Surgery.

It was therefore something of a surprise to be called in and offered the post. I accepted with alacrity. Jim Bourke joined me outside and we went out to lunch. I said to him that I had been taken aback by the lack of questions during the interview. 'Oh,' he replied, 'your real interview was yesterday afternoon.' I was thrilled to get the job and felt that at last I was making some real headway in my career.

There was a lot to do to organise to move the family from Edinburgh down to Nottingham in the six weeks that were available. We wanted to get Jake into a new school for the beginning of the spring term as he was exhibiting some signs of being a slow learner already, particularly when it came to reading.

Muriel and I went down and started to look at houses in October 1973. We were both were tired of living in the centre of Edinburgh and concentrated on villages to the north of the city towards Southwell, within acceptable travelling distance. Muriel wanted to have a place with stabling at, or very near, the house. We came across a cottage in the village of Bleasby, owned by two elderly sisters who were fanatic gardeners, with stabling as well as a garage. They put it up for auction and we were very lucky to get it. We still had to sell in Edinburgh, and as this was to be a normal sale it took a bit longer and we had a nail-biting time while we owned two houses.

CHAPTER FOURTEEN

Lecturer in Surgery: Nottingham, 1973–1977

I STARTED WORK in Nottingham on 1 December 1973 as Lecturer/Senior Registrar on the Professorial Surgical Unit, in Beeston Ward at Nottingham General Hospital. It was on the second top floor of a new tower block and had the 'modern' concept of small rooms with from one to six beds in each. This gave more privacy and flexibility of sex distribution than a Nightingale ward but it took more staff to care for the patients to the same degree, and there was no ability to take extra patients.

Jim Bourke was in charge of the day to day running of the Unit. There was no Registrar on the Unit but an SHO and two housemen who, in those days, came from one of the London Hospitals as the first cohort of Nottingham students had just started on the wards and were still nearly two years away from graduation.

The theatre suite, for some reason only known to the architect, was on the top floor of the tower block. Below us were two other surgical wards and the Pathology Laboratory. On the ground floor was the hospital kitchen and the staff canteen. This was only one catering facility for all grades and types of hospital 'workers'. It was hopeless for clinical staff because if a bleep went off in the food queue the hapless person lost his/her place and had to start again at the end of the queue.

Of some architectural interest in the older part of the hospital was a round tower containing some Medical wards with the beds placed round the outside of the circle like the hours on a clock. I have not seen or heard of any others like this.

I lived in hospital accommodation behind the hospital in 'The Park'. We had been lucky in selling the house in Edinburgh quickly and got £18,500 for it, an 85 per cent increase over the purchase price only two years previously. The completion date was 17 December and so the family moved south again, and into Fisherman's Cottage, Bleasby, the week before Christmas.

Fisherman's had started life as an ale house. It was a long, and narrow, with a staircase at each end. The only way from one end to the other was through the dining room on the ground floor, or through the guest bedroom on the first floor. The front door on to the main road, the original pub entrance, was rarely used and everyone used the back door into the kitchen.

The garden was a mixture of fruit and vegetables with a small orchard at the bottom. Separating it from the next door cottage was a walled garden in the corner of which was a large fig tree. Next door was Mrs Baggaley, an artist, and two along were the Deacons, David (a British Airways Captain) and Lynn (a nurse), who had children of the same age as ours and with whom we became close friends.

We discovered, only after we had moved in, that many senior medical staff lived either in Bleasby or in the villages on either side. Professor Hardcastle, and one of the other Consultant Surgeons, lived at the other end of the village. I don't think they believed me when I said I did not know this when we bought Fisherman's.

The village school was at that end of the village and Jake settled in well. A few days later he came home full of smiles with books that he started to read. He apparently believed, in Edinburgh, that he had to learn every word separately and felt that this was too much like hard work. His new teacher explained that there were only 26 letters in the alphabet and that all words were made up from them. He never looked back with his reading, nor his interest in learning, although his general laid-back nature (laziness) was to catch up with him again later.

The Stag was soon to prove too expensive with rising petrol prices so we rationalised our transport. I chose for economy and bought a Citroen Dyane (the swish version of the 2CV) and a new red Volvo estate for the family. The MGTC, which had lain in the garage of No. 9 was brought down and occupied the garage at Fisherman's. The children remember that they sat in the back of it, with Garth, outside the local pub, the Coach and Horses, with lemonade and a packet of crisps.

The Coach and Horses was, and probably still is, where everything in the village gets sorted. George and Mary Hall were the landlords and were also good friends. We still exchange Christmas cards. It was in the days when beer drinkers all had their own mug hanging above the bar that would be taken down and filled as the owner approached, a tradition ruined by today's health scares.

I still had to live in 1 in 3 nights when we were on call as the main Casualty department was at the General. We admitted a large number of road accidents and some of the injuries were severe. On two occasions I caused major upset by taking patients with multiple injuries straight to theatre to try to save them, not realising that they had not yet been formally admitted to the hospital. They both died on the operating table and then there was all hell to pay because of the absence of admission paperwork. On the occasions when I have done this and the patients have survived, there has been no reciprocal expression of praise, nor complaint, from those same authorities for my actions. Things, I know, have got twenty times worse in the NHS since those days.

Early in 1974 I went to the City Hospital to work with Professor Blamey in the Breast Clinic. I had the (dubious) honour of being the first Senior Registrar in Surgery in the Hospital. This caused some disquiet among the three Registrars who had had been able to organise things to suit themselves. Much more difficult was my relationship with the Consultant who shared the unit with Prof Blamey, Mr Masterman.

He was nearly 65 and about to retire in a few months. He did not approve of pethidine nor of intravenous infusions, and insisted that his patients had rectal tap water instilled by a rubber tube. We would take down the IV drip and stop pethidine by the time he did a ward round. He taught me to do partial gastrectomies for both ulcers and cancer, using a technique that I used for the rest of my own career. I came to the conclusion that a surgeon was no longer at his best once over the age of 62 or 63. I was to have this confirmed again over the years and determined that I would retire before this happened to me.

Part of my job at the City, apart from the teaching commitment, was to set up a Chemotherapy service in the Breast Clinic. This was also to evaluate different drugs and regimes of treatment. Initially we only treated recurrent, or advanced, disease and when word of this clinic got around I got referrals from all round the Region.

The non-Surgical Consultants, especially the senior ones, had a hard time accepting my clinical opinion if one was asked of the Professorial Unit. The direct referrals to me in the out-patient clinic produced a complaint that I was not a 'Consultant'. I was pleased when Roger reassured everyone that I was simply his representative and he was still the named clinician who was legally responsible.

I did not get involved with transplantation which was handled by Christine Evans. I have to describe her as 'a character' because that was what she was. There were few women in Surgery in those days and even fewer in Academic Surgery so that she had to be able to stand up to and rise above many difficulties. I got on well with her and she had a sense of humour that carried her through many a male dominated situation.

Jim, Tom, Christine and I used to gather at the Ballrace Warren pub not far from the General Hospital. The first time Jack Hardcastle came with us he asked her if she would like a half pint of beer. Christine drank beer as much, and as quickly, as Jim but she smiled and said that she did not recognise anything less than a pint as a measure of beer.

I spent a lot of time writing my thesis as I wanted to get it finished and also knew that its acceptance might be vital to me getting a good Teaching Hospital Consultant post. I did all the draft typing myself and as I knew of one person who had the one and only copy of his thesis stolen from his desk kept a total of four carbon paper copies in different locations.

I gave a summary paper of my research at the Surgical Research Society and my view that there was no value in further work on Prolactin in breast cancer at this stage. I was lucky in that I had few questions and none that I could not handle. I later attended two meetings, one in Denmark, where similar conclusions were presented and on neither occasion was my earlier original work quoted. It seemed an awful waste of valuable time and money to repeat negative findings.

The Chemotherapy clinic became well known and I as a result I became heavily involved with the drug companies who were looking for clinics who could use the next generation of drugs in clinical trials. There were some drugs that were interesting but had little or no relevance to breast cancer so that we started a second clinic to treat other adult solid tumours such as colon, stomach and pancreas.

We were referred many terminally ill patients who were desperate for any chance of 'cure'. I was distressed to find that a number of them had not even been told the true diagnosis and we made it a condition of referral that their own Consultant had to break the news to them before I would see them. Many of the patients had such advanced disease that it was not a fair trial of the drugs.

A new group of drugs, BCNU and CCNU, were very toxic and could only be given once a week as a tablet. Even so the results were disappointing and many of the general side effects of chemotherapy were severe, making their use inappropriate. A few years later a doctor used them to murder his wife by causing severe agranulocytosis (low white cells). I was ahead of police thinking when a copy of the prescription appeared in the newspapers showing a daily, not weekly, dose.

We treated most patients referred on the grounds that if we did not try we would never succeed. On that basis we had a number of anecdotally spectacular successes, so much so that we were repeatedly asking the pathologists to review the slides of some tumours to confirm that we were actually dealing with cancer. This occasionally caused wrath among our pathology colleagues who thought that we were doubting their diagnostic skills. This was an early example of pathology audit which has now become headline news.

These experiences left me with the view that it was necessary to treat all cancers aggressively if there was to be any chance of curing some patients. At the same time I began to ask myself what was the correct definition of 'cure' when it came to cancer?

One of the first extraordinary cases of long-term response to treatment was an ex-policeman who was sent to me with pancreatic cancer. He had been 17 stone but arrived in the clinic on a stretcher weighing less than 7 stone and looking terminally ill. Even I was reluctant to treat him and we had a long discussion and in the end agreed to try. He responded to the treatment, and went back to about 15 stone and work as a security guard. We still exchange Christmas cards and John Wordsley and his wife May have visited me in the North on a couple of occasions.

At the City there were a number of other specialist units. One of the foremost was Gastroenterology with Mike Langman who was the Professor of Therapeutics. He was a very colourful character and of the 'modern' breed of Professors wearing flamboyant clothes and ties, and mixing with the junior staff in the pub. We did the endoscopic work for them and had a very good working relationship.

There was a large Gynaecology Unit in which, at one stage, worked Mr Rodney Ledward. Recently there was a high profile investigation into his clinical practice. He was described as a flamboyant character and he certainly was, even in those days, but I remember him as having a fairly good clinical judgement and being a good operator. I was thus surprised at recent events.

Another surgical trainee, Chris Ingoldby, passed through the unit and recently his clinical skills and judgement have also been questioned. A third colleague from those days, who became well known in the media, was Richard Arnot. It was in his flat in Saudi Arabia that the fateful party was being held when a nurse fell to her death in mysterious circumstances.

On moving to Nottingham I went on to List 4 in the Naval Reserve. This means that the only commitment is the two weeks annual training. I had heard through the grapevine that the RNR was establishing a

Surgical Support Team, similar to the M*A*S*H unit, but strictly an all male staff in those days. I wrote to its Commanding Officer, Tom Bucknell with the London Division, but found out that all his slots were filled. A second unit was forming based on the other Naval Hospital in Plymouth and so I approached them directly.

I was keen to get involved with this Unit especially with my Marine background but I was also frustrated that at the age of 37 I had been a Surgeon Lieutenant for a long time. To be the Surgical Specialist for the SST I thought that I should be up a rank. A little to my surprise the Admiralty accepted this reasoning and also backdated the seniority by a year. They did tick me off, however, for dealing with them direct and not through my Unit; which was technically still in Edinburgh.

The first exercise of the SST was held on Salisbury Plain, using tented accommodation, at the end of October 1974. I think there was only one other member of the team who was Commando trained and it came as a shock to them to be living rough in the late autumn. We taught the inexperienced members about living in the field, some defence tactics and camouflage. This latter was so successful that we were nearly all squashed one night when a troop of tanks drove into, and through, our camp without seeing us.

We clinicians slipped out of the camp down to the local pub where I introduced the others to scrumpy. The landlord would only allow us half a pint at a time, it was so strong. My 'scrumpy befuzzed arithmetic' let me down when we were challenged by the sentry on the numerical pass-code. We then spent the rest of the night in the makeshift guard-house, much to everyone's amusement.

The first students at the City Hospital decided to put on a Christmas Pantomime. They were well into rehearsals when they lost the services of the person who was going to do the lighting and sound. They approached me and, after some consideration and studying the script, I agreed to give it a go. I was surprised how easily it all came back to me after something like fifteen years. I had no difficulty in following the script and my main concern was in getting two blackouts, which fitted with a sound one, exactly instantaneous.

After a full year in Bleasby we felt really at home and were enjoying village life. We made a lot of friends there and Muriel began to spend more time with horses. She had met Angela Eastwood who was also 'into horses'. She was German, married to Bill, and her father had been a regular officer in the Panzer Corps at the invasion of Poland in 1939. He was a very interesting man to talk to and I believed him when he said that it was many years before the majority of the population realised exactly what Hitler was up to. He pointed out that it was the Army who tried, and failed, to get rid of him.

I had had to become a gardener and although I knew precious little about it found that I really enjoyed pottering about and learning as I went. Nottingham, being in the middle of the country, is warmer than many places and consequently more exotic plants will grow there, even outdoors. One disadvantage is that it is as far from the sea as you can get in England so I got little sailing.

In the summer of 1975 we agreed to go back to Tamarui with the crowd as it was not too far a drive to the ferry at Portsmouth. We took the boat and Lisa, a friend's daughter, as a sort of au-pair to help look after the children. This time when we arrived the boat was on its mooring within an hour.

The intermingling of couples, and skinny dipping at midnight, was even more in evidence this time and at least once Muriel came back in a high state of sexual arousal. What had been going on I did not know but could guess. In the light of my own affair I was not in any position to do other than accept it as there was no suggestion that it was interfering with the marriage, as was our agreement.

I elected to do a year in Urology, another of the specialist subjects at the City. The senior Urologist was a lovely man, Matt Grey, who was also about to retire at 65. He was becoming a little forgetful but otherwise was still full of beans and was a good teacher. Having done Urology previously I only had a short learning curve on the much newer and clearer fibre-optic instruments.

The other consultant was Patrick Bates who was very young, full of energy and ideas, but just a little eccentric. He was interested in total cystectomy as a treatment for bladder cancer with the replacement of the bladder by an ileal loop into which the ureters are implanted. It is a very 'stressful' operation for the patient and I noticed that in the cases where it was not possible to remove the bladder, but only do the diversion, the patients fared much better post-operatively. We demonstrated that we could reverse the serious protein loss after the operation by feeding the patients intravenously for a few days before the operation, and again after it.

Patrick Bates had taken me through the operation a number of times and suggested I start one case with the Registrar. He would come in time to take me through the second stage. All went well and I completed the first stage but there was no sign of him. I was getting worried about not getting the operation finished and asked someone to phone his home. His eight-year-old daughter answered. We managed to elicit from her that he had gone down the road to a neighbour's house and that she would go down and tell him we wanted him. He had completely forgotten about the operation.

We saw, and operated on, some very large kidney tumours. Like the thoracic surgery before, one has to learn not to be afraid of mastering special techniques not normally used in General Surgery. In renal surgery it is vascular techniques that are needed to allow opening and closing of the large veins, such as the Vena Cave, which may mean the difference between eradicating the tumour and leaving a bit behind. The really sad cases were in children with huge Wilms tumours that sometimes were removable and sometimes not. Even when they did come out there was always the risk that they had seeded to the lungs and the operation would turn out to have been in vain.

Another trainee who joined us at this time was a young Scottish Registrar called Ken Queen. He was married to Midge (Margaret) and they had both worked in the 'Gate' at Glasgow Royal Infirmary. Midge became one of the Sisters in Casualty at the General. We became very good friends indeed.

We were always being asked to go to other parts of the hospital to pass catheters, usually in men. This happened when the junior staff had tried and failed. We had a policy that they should not continue to try but to call us. If we failed at one attempt we would take the patient to theatre and pass it under local, or occasionally general, anaesthesia.

One Friday evening at about 5 p.m. I was called to a female geriatric ward to pass a catheter. I assumed that the nurses and the house-person had tried and went prepared to find a problem. In fact a nurse had tried and asked the 'doctor' to try but as she was 'going off for the weekend', this doctor had told them to call me. I blew my top at this but passed the old lady's catheter, easily, before going in search of this doctor who had not yet escaped from the hospital. This was the first time I had encountered the militant working of the young doctors that has gone on getting worse ever since.

In September 1975 I got the opportunity to be involved in a Surgical Support Team exercise when the Admiralty asked for volunteers for a two week period. All that we were supposed to know was that we had to arrive at Swindon railway station by a certain time on 14 September. It was easy to find out that the Commando Units and Carriers were going to be in the Med.

We flew out to Malta and on arrival were taken straight to a Landing Ship Logistics (LSL) that was waiting specially for us, all the other ships having already left. We were ushered off the plane and into a bus without entering the airport terminal and were on the ship forty minutes later. For many years when asked if I had been to Malta, I would enjoy saying, 'Yes, but only for forty minutes.'

We sailed to the Gulf of Soros which is in European, as opposed to Asian, Turkey. It is on the western side of the infamous Gallipoli peninsula. The fleet was preparing for an amphibious landing of 3 Commando Brigade. We landed as part of Commando Logistics Regiment and set up the SST just inland from the beach. We had no sooner put the first ward tent up than it was filled with twenty real casualties. Luckily none was serious, the worst being a Marine whose foot had got trapped in the door of a landing craft, but his boots had prevented more than bad bruising.

I was the only Commando trained person in the team and upset some of the others by disappearing while they struggled to get the SST and our own living accommodation erected. I was finding things like chairs and tables, and negotiating for our tent to be included in the mains electrical circuit that the engineers would be laying, to give us light and to make our life bearable.

The whole of the Regiment was living on hard rations that could be supplemented with local purchase, if any was found. The next day I set off, found a vegetable patch and then some local fishermen. I negotiated, in cigarettes, for fresh vegetables and fish. The vegetables were delivered immediately, in a wheelbarrow, but there was no sign of any fish until the third day when a small fishing boat pulled up on our beach full of fish, more than enough to feed everyone.

We did a major casualty reception exercise using twenty Midshipmen 'volunteers'. This was mainly a test of the paperwork, and the physical movement of casualties. We practised Triage that caused an upset among those Midshipmen who were deemed non-saveable and put outside the back of the tent. They had been sent ashore with only a bottle of water and a pack of sandwiches for their 24-hour ordeal. Being in some credit with the cooks I arranged for them to be fed with the rest of us. This turned a sullen bunch of young men into a group who were good fun.

One night some bright spark (pun) pushed a lit thunder-flash under the edge of the tent right next to my head. I woke and realised what it was, got hold of the blunt end and had just got it back out of the tent and let go of it when it went off before the edge of the tent came down again. I suffered superficial burns to the hand but the skin was not broken. The flash blinded me for a couple of hours and this caused me, and the hierarchy in the Unit, a severe panic. I was annoyed but I received a roundabout apology from the perpetrator that it had not been aimed at me personally. Five years later my experience helped a soldier in a much worse incident.

The non-medical members were taken out on a 'patrol' by the RSM. I had recovered from my injury and decided to have a game with them. I took out the other clinicians on 'patrol' to see if I could ambush the first as it returned to the camp. I took a calculated gamble as to the route he would lead them back, through the dunes, to the camp and lay in wait for them at that spot. Just when I thought I had been wrong and the others were champing to return to camp I heard them approaching.

Arriving at the spot I had chosen the RSM stopped them and I heard him say, 'This is the place that I would have intercepted you if I was part of the defence team.' Standing up I said, 'I'm pleased all my training has not been wasted, RSM.' I thought we were going to have to resuscitate him but having regained his composure he congratulated me on the interception. This did our reputation, as a Reserve Unit, no harm at all and indeed to have pulled one on the RSM gained us a lot of kudos. He himself was full of praise, and he and I became good friends over the next years.

At the end of our week ashore we were to be replaced by the Regular SST that had sailed out on HMS *Hermes*, the Commando Carrier (as she was then). The rotation was to be done by helicopter using two Wessex 5s. None of the team had done this sort of thing before so the RSM and I practised the drill with them several times.

On the day itself they did the boarding and un-boarding, with their kit, as if they had been doing it every day and when we got off on the Carrier – most hadn't been on one before – they were congratulated for their efficiency by the deck crew who had obviously been warned about these 'novices'.

One serious problem was that all our heavy kit was still on the LSL, at anchor some miles away. To me there was only one way to go and get it and that was by Wessex. This was not the view held by the tasking team who were not going to release a slot for such an 'unimportant' task. I decided it was time to chat up the Squadron and went in search of their Senior Pilot who I knew from the old days. I put the problem to him and he spoke to the CO.

The solution was simple. They did a mail round to all the ships twice a day. They would take two of us out in the morning to collect the gear together and pick us, and the luggage, up on the afternoon run. It went like clockwork and must have taken no more than two minutes extra on their schedule to recover it for us. Our team was delighted and the remainder of the Wardroom puzzled as to how we had done it.

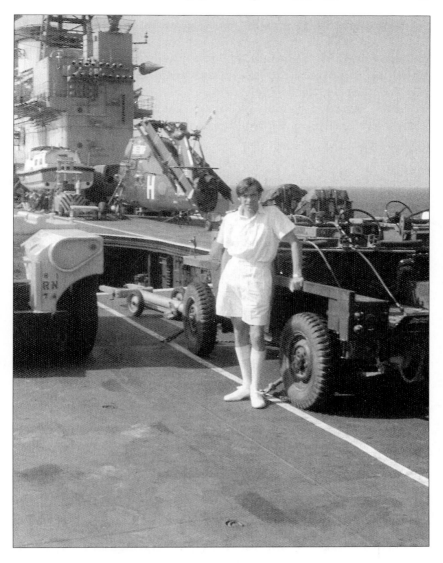

HMS *Hermes* in the Bosphorus, 1975.

Hermes then sailed up the Sea of Marmara to Istanbul where we anchored in the main stream of the Bosphorus. Getting ashore, and back, was a hazardous affair. A barge was moored alongside, the ship's boats came alongside it and one jumped at a suitable moment. There was a fearsome current racing through from the Black Sea and it was quite choppy. I don't think if anyone had fallen in they would have survived.

We managed to spend some time sightseeing and visited the Blue Mosque, the Souk (market) and saw some belly dancing. What was very noticeable was the complete lack of any adherence to normal road rules. Cars, and especially taxis, went the wrong way on dual carriageways and paid not the slightest attention to red traffic lights. I have subsequently warned a number of people going to Turkey about the traffic light problem and advised them not to hire a car under any circumstances.

On the Saturday we were due to fly home but the aircraft that was tasked for us broke down, in Cyprus, on the way out. The RAF, as I have commented before, have some strange habits and one is to keep the load allocated to that aircraft and do not use the aircraft in sequence. We were sent back to the ship and were told that it would be Monday, at the earliest, before we would get away.

Everyone in the party had to be back at work on the Monday morning, and some, like me, had a long journey in UK to get home. We pointed out that our Recall orders ran out at midnight on the Sunday and asked who was going to be responsible if anything untoward happened to any of us after that hour, or who was going to try to find anyone at MoD to extend our orders on a Saturday evening?

Some sensible person put us on a Hercules that night. We flew back, overnight, via Cyprus where we refuelled and then on along the Mediterranean, turning right at Sicily and up the coast of Italy and directly across Europe to UK. It was a very long flight as the 'Herk' is not very fast but is very noisy. Going to the toilet was an experience as the Elsan is housed in the rear of the plane so that one has to walk on the tailgate, over thin air, to get to it. We all got home in time to go to work as normal on the Monday.

At about this time there was a move to have a strike, or a go slow, among doctors over pay. I went to the meeting as the most senior non-consultant surgeon in the hospital but I found myself being told to refrain from commenting, or to leave the meeting, as I was not an NHS employee but a University one. Sadly there has been a pay differential between NHS and University clinical staffs ever since. There was a motion from the psychiatrists, the largest group at the meeting, to work to rule. Matt Grey, to the delight of the gathering, suggested that this would mean that the psychiatrists would actually have to do more if they were working to contract. Hoots of mirth all round.

Mike Metcalf joined the team at the City and he also had a Citroen 2CV and lived in Burton Joyce, on my way home to Bleasby. We sometimes met at his local pub after work and, as the car park was usually empty at that time, would drive round it up on two wheels as demonstrated in the Citroen adverts.

Mike, also a Scottish graduate, was married to Jane, an anaesthetist. Of all my friends over the years he has been the one with the worst of all luck. Jane had twins and they lost one soon after birth. He and Jane split up some years later at about the time he got a Consultant post in Whitehaven, near Carlisle. He remarried a few years later and soon afterwards he had a massive and almost fatal stroke, which has left him severely handicapped.

After nearly two years at the City I moved back to the General. Jim Bourke was doing a study of the time taken off work by Nottinghamshire miners after an inguinal hernia repair. It was quite usual for them to be off work for three months although there was no scientific evidence to support this time. He divided the patients into two groups, one taking three months off and the other returning to work when we said it was clinically safe, and the patient wanted to.

We found that the men were happy to go back sooner rather than later, after about six weeks, but soon ran up against the National Union of Mineworkers who accused us of denying their members their fundamental right to three months off. They only backed down when asked to produce documentary evidence to substantiate this claim.

Prof. Hardcastle, with his interest in small bowel function, had a programme for the surgical treatment of morbid obesity. We were dealing with patients, mainly ladies, of 22 stones or more. They were expected to have tried all the other types of forced weight loss including having their jaws wired together and have been pronounced 'normal' by a psychiatrist.

We did about twenty of these although by the end only the Professor was still keen on the idea. We were finally convinced that we were wasting our time when we discovered that one of the ladies had been a champion fish and chip eater in her home town of Grantham. Now she could eat till the cows came home she had retaken the title.

For a lot of these procedures we had the services of the new Professor of Anaesthetics who was interested in the type of anaesthesia where the patient was kept very light but felt no sensation of pain. This was in later years to get a bad reputation because it was almost impossible to know the level of consciousness of the patient and consequently there were a number of cases of litigation when the patient maintained that they had been awake and aware all the time.

My first experience of this came one night when I had to take an elderly patient to theatre for an emergency procedure. I had just finished the operation when a hand appeared around the drapes and proceeded to scratch the open wound. We applied some local antibiotic powder to the wound and, luckily, he did not get a wound infection.

The petrol crisis of two years previously had forced down the price of collectors' cars and I had been waiting for the right moment to buy a MG TF, which we had had in Singapore. I saw an advertisement for a red one that had been rebuilt by experts and had the registration number 1954 MG. The asking price was only slightly more than the previous owner had spent on the rebuild. I have kept her with me ever since and still use it every summer.

That summer we went back to Denmark in the new red Volvo OAL 147M. We drove across country to Harwich. In those days it was a truly cross-country drive and I underestimated how long it would take with the result that we very nearly missed the ferry. There was a very high stress level in the car by the time we got there.

Jake was nine and Fiona six at this stage. The beach outside the summerhouse had become a nudist beach and as there were very few people about we also went out in the nude. That is until the children wanted to go swimming when they insisted, in their own logic, on donning swimming costumes while in the water. On one occasion our naked elderly gentleman neighbour came across and offered Muriel some strawberries, or raspberries, while standing directly over her. I was hugely amused but I think she was just seriously embarrassed.

I settled into doing my RNR fortnight in the autumn each year and this year I was asked if I could do a locum at RNH Haslar in Portsmouth. The Navy uses the old system of hierarchy in medicine by having Surgical Specialists but only the senior one was a Consultant. I qualified for this junior position, being a fairly senior senior-registrar. Haslar is, being the centre of Naval Medicine, a little snooty and pompous and this came through to me, as a Reservist, when dealing with certain people.

As always on these trips the locum is on call for the middle weekend from about noon on the Friday till Monday morning. There is not usually a lot to do but on this occasion I had hardly finished my lunch when I was bleeped to go the Officers' ward. I found a patient with a dehisced (burst) wound. He had had his upper abdominal incisional hernia repaired only that morning.

I took him back to theatre to find, a little to my surprise, that his hernia had been repaired with a single layer of not very strong, continuous nylon thread. I did a 'proper' Mayo repair of three layers of interrupted strong nylon and put tension stitches in at the end for added strength. There was a real sting in the tail with this case as he turned out to be the First Officer of the *QE2* and was due to sail in a few days, in charge, as the Captain was on leave. I was not popular when I pointed out that that was Cunard's problem; and that of my colleague who had done the first repair of the day.

Later that day I was summoned back to the Officers' ward to see another patient. I think, in retrospect, that this was due to them finding 'my metal' with the first case. I was ushered into a private room housing a crusty old seadog Admiral of the Fleet, Knight of the Realm. There was a strong smell of gangrene in the air. He was in a wheelchair and had already lost one leg.

He demanded to know who I was, what my qualifications were and why was I there in his room. I explained that the nurses were concerned about his foot and that they wanted me to look at it, but if he didn't I would go away again. This floored him a bit and he grudgingly got on top of the bed with help from the nurses who then took down the stinking dressing.

His whole foot had wet gangrene and the blue ischaemia went well up the lower leg. I told him the time had come to part with this one as well before the sepsis got into the bloodstream and finished him off.

'When?' he demanded.

'The sooner the better. As soon as we can get theatre organised,' I replied. 'You have to agree and sign the consent form and I will do it immediately. You will feel much better afterwards.'

He looked me straight in the eye and said, 'You'd better be right, Doc.'

'I am,' I replied.

'Please go and explain it all to my wife,' he said.

I went out and talked to her Ladyship who was a lovely gentle lady, quite unlike her husband. I explained what I had just told the Admiral and that he was a little taken aback at me being a reservist. 'Thank you,' she said. 'No one here has had the courage to tell him because of who he is. Please carry on and do what is needed.'

We found the most senior anaesthetist we could that weekend and I removed his leg with a second above knee amputation that evening. I gave him a large dose of antibiotic to prevent any systemic sepsis and went to bed that night with my fingers firmly crossed. I realised the gravity of my position if I lost the Admiral while in my care over the weekend.

The following morning when I went to the ward in fear and trepidation, I found the Admiral sitting in his wheelchair reading the paper. He was gracious enough, in his own gruff way, to thank me and agreed with me that he felt much better without his 'rotten' leg. Her Ladyship was again her charming self and thanked me profusely for my kindness and understanding. 'He's not the easiest person to talk to,' she said.

'No,' I replied, 'but I think he and I understand each other.'

A 206 (Officer's appraisal form) is filled in by the Medical Officer in Charge after such an attachment by a Reservist. The Officer concerned does not get to see it unless it is an adverse one in which case it is mandatory for him/her to see it. When I left Haslar on this occasion, I was given a typed form signed by the Surgeon Captain MOIC which in essence was a reference and read, 'A pleasant and very able general surgeon who has been a considerable asset to the hospital during his two week training period.'

Reading between the lines I detected not a small input from the Admiral because I'm quite sure that Cunard didn't feel the same way. For some years after this locum I was repeatedly invited to rejoin the Navy as a Consultant and although tempted on a number of the occasions I never did sign on.

On my return to Nottingham, I had a priority of getting my thesis finished and bound. I had let Professor Forrest see my final draft and he felt that it was sufficiently good to be accepted. One of the girls in the department office typed the final copy, I got it to the binders in the late autumn and submitted to Aberdeen University in October.

It was a sad year for Muriel as her mother, who had been ill for some time with advanced breast cancer, died. We went up to Aberdeen for the funeral which, like all funerals, was a truly depressing and upsetting event.

With nearly three years completed in the Senior Registrar Grade I felt it was now time to start applying for jobs. I was now 39 and definitely long in the tooth to be getting a prime Consultant job. There were two options open to me. One was to continue to pursue an academic path and get a Senior Lecturer post. I had never seen myself as a Professor of Surgery, for very many reasons, but Jack Hardcastle felt otherwise and was keen for me to go this way. At the time there was only one vacancy that would have suited my career and that was at Charing Cross Hospital in London.

I had prided myself that I had got on reasonably well in Surgery without ever having done a job in London and had no desire to change now. I also would not have got on with the person in charge of the Breast Unit there. Finally, not wanting to hold a Chair, it would have meant a further move into an NHS Consultant post in three to five years time.

My own choice was to go for a Teaching Hospital job in the first instance, hopefully with an interest in cancer. The British Association of Surgical Oncology had just been established and I was a founder member, firmly believing that this was the way forward if patients were to get a holistic approach to the management of their cancers. Failing this, and I was going to allow myself a year to achieve it, I would go for a non-teaching hospital job in either General Surgery or Urology.

A job came up in Leicester that Jack Hardcastle suggested I apply for. It would have been possible to do the job without moving from Fisherman's; just. I felt I was well placed to get the job, the main competition coming from their own Senior Registrar, whom I knew quite well. When we arrived for the interview we were presented with a piece of paper stating that the job description had been altered and that experience in paediatric surgery was required. This immediately ruled me out but I went ahead with the interview for the experience.

I was angry when they offered the job to the local candidate who I knew had no more experience in paediatric surgery than I. They had fiddled the situation by arranging for him to go for this specialist training after he had been given the job. I was so incensed that I threatened to complain to the College about the way it had been set up. Jack Hardcastle persuaded me not to and I suppose in retrospect that he was right.

The second job was in Newcastle upon Tyne, a city that I had only passed through in the train, or when catching a ferry to Scandinavia. They specifically asked for a Surgical Oncologist to set up a Breast Clinic in the city. I applied and was confident I would get strong backing from not only my current bosses, but also my previous ones in the subject.

I was short-listed and invited for interview on 11 November 1976. I went up to Newcastle before this to look round and meet as many people involved with the job as possible. I thought the post was ideal for my plans as it was based at the General Hospital (the old workhouse), which also housed the Radiotherapy and Oncology Centre.

To my dismay I learned that they too had a strong local candidate who had been on a sabbatical in Canada and who had come home especially for the interview. It was with some surprise, therefore, that I learned that he had withdrawn his application on the morning of the interview, having accepted a job in Bath.

There was a formidable panel at the interview including Professor Johnston, the Professor of Surgery, Chris Venables, Mr Smydie (who had failed me in the London exam), Mr McEwan, the well known oesophageal surgeon from Darlington, and various University representatives. It was a gruelling interview but to my intense relief and amazement, I was offered the post. I accepted with alacrity and agreed to start on 1 March 1977.

Mr Venables then took me across to the Unit to meet 'the team' and we were outraged to find out that during the course of the interviews the hospital authorities had closed one of the wards because of a shortage of nurses. We were not to know it at the time but this was only a foretaste of things to come over the subsequent years.

Muriel and I now faced moving yet again but felt that we had adequate time on this occasion. We had not made allowance for the crash in house prices and would be lucky to sell the house without a loss.

I was in theatre one day at Christmas 1976 when I became aware of a pair of blue eyes watching me over a mask. The eyes were quite disturbing and belonged to a tall, slim, mature, 3rd year student nurse called Judi. She had trained to be a teacher and had taught in London's East End for a year or two, before deciding it was not for her. She later worked on Beeston Ward and I got to know her better.

Fate then took a hand. Bill and Angela Eastwood had been asked to a Christmas party and invited Muriel and me along. The party was in a large country house in Long Eaton, south-west of the city. I was completely floored when the door was opened by the daughter of the house, the girl with the blue eyes. We did not have a chance to speak to each other much during the evening but I could feel the 'vibes' between us. As we were leaving she asked if she would be seeing me again since I was leaving Nottingham soon and I asked her if she wanted to. She replied, 'Yes.' I only did see her once more, socially, before I left Nottingham.

I got a letter in the middle of January from Aberdeen University to say that my thesis had been accepted subject to ten spelling and punctuation corrections. I was delighted that this was out of the way before I started my Consultant post in Newcastle.

It is only two and a half hours by fast car from Bleasby to Newcastle so Muriel and I travelled north to look at houses. I replaced the Citroen with another TR6, this time a second-hand yellow one, for the travelling to come.

We bought Ordnance Survey maps of the whole area and I drew five and ten mile circles on them. We were torn between living in the countryside, or in a more urban environment. In the case of the former the best area seemed to be south-west of the city but at that time this lovely countryside was covered with a layer of iron ore dust from the Consett Steel Works. On the urban side there were few places where the horses could be accommodated except in Darras Hall, a satellite town north of the city.

We had had no luck selling Fisherman's and as March approached it became clear that we would probably have to leave the move until after the end of the summer school term in June to move up to the North East and became resigned to a likely separation of three to four months.

We had several farewell parties both in the Hospitals and in the village. For some reason people must have got the idea that I was a beer drinker because I was given a pair of pewter tankards with 'Bleasby' and the dates engraved on them.

In the last few weeks in the village the river Trent, which was half a mile away, flooded to such an extent that the water came right up the road to the cottage next door. Barbara Baggaley, the artist next door, painted two lovely watercolours of Fisherman's, one viewed from the main street and the other a group of three sketches of the back and the outbuildings. They are now hanging in my dining room. It was certainly one of the nicest houses we lived in.

CHAPTER FIFTEEN

Newcastle: Darras Hall, 1977–1980

I STARTED as a Consultant General Surgeon, with an interest in Oncology, on Tuesday 1 March 1977. The surgical block at Newcastle General was a three-storey brick building. The four surgical wards were Nightingale type wards, the kind that I found very easy to work, although there could be a lack of privacy for patients if the nursing and medical staff were not carefully considerate. I shared wards 17 and 18 on the ground floor with Chris Venables, a Senior Lecturer. As a Trauma hospital the General had an Intensive Care Unit, a Coronary Care Unit, and a High Dependency Unit in the Regional Neurology and Neurosurgical Unit that were on the site.

A novel feature of our unit, before they became the 'in thing' in the NHS, was the presence of five Day-case beds on the top floor. They were invaluable for relieving the in-patient beds of minor operations. The remainder of the top floor was an orthopaedic and casualty ward. The Casualty Surgeon was David Milne who had taught me Anatomy. Dick Madeley, from my medical class year, was the Professor of Virology.

On my first visit to a local pub, I discovered that the 'Geordies' have an entirely different attitude to drinking from the rest of Britain. They seem to believe that the supply of beer or lager is about to dry up and order the next drink when the previous one is only half consumed. This means that everyone has two glasses on the go at the same time. I thought that the Nottingham miners drank a lot.

I operated all day on Mondays and had a wonderful anaesthetist called Katie Clarke. She got to know my obsession with punctuality and would get the first patient ready to anaesthetise for my arrival. I always spoke to my patients in the anaesthetic room. I felt that this gave the patients confidence and also allowed me to confirm with them what it was I was about to do to them, and which side, if there were two or more.

I never allowed any junior to operate on a patient unless they had seen them in the ward beforehand, and made them see them again in the anaesthetic room as I did. If they had not done these things I did not let them do the operation. In the light of some of the recent problems in Surgery I was glad I was so obsessive. Some of the juniors, especially in the latter years, never got this message.

Tuesday mornings I was in outpatients and started the Breast Clinic. It began very small and nineteen years later was enormous. That afternoon I did an Endoscopy list but in the early days this was not very satisfactory as it was done in the main theatre. If the morning list overran I had to wait to get started. Chris Venables and I agreed that this had to change and a dedicated Unit was formed.

On Wednesday I had a morning operating list and the afternoon was supposedly free but I always seemed to find something to do, one of which was to see any patients who wished to see me privately. I had had a long discussion with Colin Davidson, who had a huge private practice in Bristol, about the advisability, or not, of consulting in the Nuffield Private Hospital. He advised me not to become involved unless I was certain about it. I have nothing morally, politically or personally against private medicine but I never regretted not getting too involved.

On Thursday morning I did my general surgical outpatient clinic. This did not last my whole consultant career as the speciality breast work took over in the end. In the afternoon I did Colonoscopy, a service that was new to the hospital and to the city. On Wednesday and Friday mornings I taught the medical students.

In those great days the hospital was run by a very small group of people. There was the Medical Director, an Administrator, a Staffing officer and the Matron. Dr Richardson, a Consultant Diabetologist, was the Director, Mr Belton was the Administrator, Dorothy Trigg was his assistant and she knew everything and everyone in the hospital, and Miss Shaw was the Matron.

Each of the functional units in the hospital had a Clinician in Administrative Charge. In our case that was Alf Petty. The second week I was there I was introduced to the first of many years of after-hours meetings. The Medical Staff Committee met once a month, which all Consultants attended, as did the Sub-Division of General Surgery. The Division of Surgery met every three months.

These two systems covered the mechanisms for running the hospital service within the Hospital and the city. It worked well and was very lean on paid administrative or managerial staff. We did our clinical duties to the full and all of us put a lot of work through the hospital. By the time of my retirement nineteen years later I calculated that my in-patient through-put was down to about 60 per cent owing to loss of facilities, junior staff, beds and nurses and loss of control to a top heavy management system.

One of the first things I did when I started was to go round and visit all the departments in the hospital such as the laboratories, the X-ray department, the Casualty department and the Oncology/Radiotherapy department to introduce myself, and meet their heads of department and as many staff as possible.

Bill Ross, in charge of Radiotherapy, was very much a spade and shovel man and was, at that time, the Colonel of the local TA Field Hospital Unit based in Newcastle. He and I had a sort of love hate relationship but mostly we were able to work together. He was always the Colonel and I was always the junior as a mere Lieutenant Commander. He was succeeded as Colonel by Katie Clarke, who was the first female Colonel of this Unit.

Directly opposite one of the gates of the hospital was the Headquarters of the local Royal Marine Reserve Unit. I made an appointment to visit the Unit to meet the CO and the Principal Medical Officer, Hartly Hanson, a GP from Chester le Street. Colonel Manuel, like Captain Mainwaring of *Dad's Army*, was a banker.

I was welcomed with open arms, not just because I was Commando trained, but because Hartley had been promoted to Commander and was going to go down to the base RNR Unit on the Tyne, HMS *Colliope*, as Senior Medical Officer. The commitment at RMR Tyne was slightly more than the normal in that there was a need to provide safety cover on the ranges when the Unit went on live firing exercises. Such was the enthusiasm for my services at RMR Tyne, rather than RNR Tyne, that my transfer came through immediately and was dated 3 May 1977. I had only been in Newcastle two months.

I had my first meeting with Professor Johnston two weeks after I arrived. We had a long discussion about my proposals for the breast clinic and my views of Surgical Oncology in general. He was also a member of BASO and suggested that I stand for the National Committee and that we try to get the meeting held in Newcastle at an early date. We discussed the need to develop Mammography in Newcastle and he put me in touch with Peter Hacking, a Radiologist at the RVI. He also asked me to take over the supervision of one of the ongoing MD projects in the department. All in all I thought that it had been a good meeting.

Muriel came up house hunting and we decided that the best thing to do was to find somewhere that 'would do' in the meantime so that we could look for the ideal long-term home from a base in Newcastle. We found an old converted farm building in Darras Hall at 159

Runneymede Road, called 'The Granary'. It had a one-acre field with a
three stable block. It was however completely landlocked by other houses
on all sides. We made a bid for it as the best interim solution although
we still had had no meaningful offers for Fisherman's.

News of my move to Newcastle spread through the pharmaceutical
network in the area fast and three companies that I did a lot of work
for and who supported me well over the years were ICI, Lederle and
Lilly.

I was also lucky in that, needing a Radiotherapist with whom to work
closely, Peter Dawes had just returned to Newcastle from an attachment
to the Royal Marsden in London. He and I saw cancer therapy in a
very similar light and worked together, starting with the breast clinic,
for all the time I was working.

Muriel and the children moved up to '159' in the middle of June.
Luckily the two cottages were very much alike and the furniture fitted
well into the new one. A major drawback from my point of view, and
my growing collection of vehicles, was that there was only a tiny single
garage at the new house, into which we were already going to have to
put the freezer.

Of eighteen sets of neighbours only two were really pleasant; most
were aloof or indifferent and some were downright rude. Our immediate
neighbour up the road, a member of the Barratt family, only spoke to
me three times in the entire three years we were in the house, twice to
complain about bonfires and once that a box of wine had been delivered
to their house one Christmas. He didn't bring it round with him either.

The Granary had been a pig farm and there were still some old sties
down by the stables and two old wooden sheds up near the house. We
decided to replace the sheds with a quadruple garage and get rid of the
pig sties by burning them. We informed the fire brigade of our intentions,
and the timing, when the wind would cause least inconvenience to all
these neighbours. We told the majority of them about the plan, but not
all. It was quite a blaze and the uninformed neighbours tried, unsuccessfully, to get the fire brigade interested. We were amused because none
of those whom we had told let on to them. I felt that that was very
telling.

I sold the TR and I replaced it with a Fiat X/19, a tiny rear-engined
sports car with a targa roof (one that is a flat panel which lifts off). The
X/19 was designed as the replacement for the MG Midget, and it was
only when British Leyland did not put it into production that Fiat
bought the design.

I had a meeting with Peter Hacking who was interested in mammography and we discussed the possibility of putting a bid in for funding as part of the National Breast Screening Trial that Pat Forrest and the Government were setting up. Pat Forrest and Roger Blamey were keen for us to be involved and we wrote a protocol as requested.

The Queen Elizabeth Hospital, Gateshead, was running a Charity Breast Screening Programme using mammography and thermography. This programme, and the large number of women from both banks of the Tyne who had been screened there, led us to fail to get the funding. The statisticians had, quite rightly, come to the conclusion that we would not have a 'clean enough' sample of unscreened women.

At the General we did not have a dedicated mammogram machine but had to share a room and equipment with another investigation. I was pleased that Bill Simpson, Consultant Radiologist, was interested in the technique and we developed the diagnostic service on a shoestring.

I was also disturbed by the decision of the Professor to get John Farndon, one of the Senior Lecturers, to start a breast clinic in the RVI. John and I got on well together and had similar ideas on management of the disease so that as long as he was there we ran the two clinics in tandem. Ours, at the General, always stayed the larger, once it really got to the notice of the GPs.

At the beginning of the school year Jake went to Coates Endowed Middle School in Ponteland, which had a good reputation for a general education although it was run on comprehensive lines. All of my colleagues spoke highly of it. Fiona, who was still only seven, went to the first school in Darras Hall. They both seemed to settle in well.

Now that I was a consultant I joined the Association of Surgeons, which is the non-academic equivalent of the Surgical Research Society, and the British Society of Gastroenterology.

I learned that the 'new boy' gets all the jobs that no one really wants and the previous 'new boy' wants to give up. I found myself on the Drugs and Therapeutics Committee for the City and the Library Committee for the General. In all the years I sat on the former I do not recall we achieved anything useful and in the latter we seemed only to rubber stamp ideas put forward by the Librarian.

In the October I was invited by Pat Forrest to give a presentation on my Chemotherapy work to the British Breast Group which he had founded a few years previously. I was very delighted when Pat Forrest and Roger Blamey told me they were going to put me forward for membership but it took two attempts for me to be accepted.

Out of the blue one day my secretary rang through to say that there was a phone call for me from Nottingham. I assumed that it would be

Jim, or another colleague, but it turned out to be Judi. I had only seen her once since leaving Nottingham when I was down for a meeting. She was coming north to stay with one of her friends in Sunderland. My feelings were very mixed. On the one hand I was excited at the prospect but on the other was aware where such a meeting might lead. I did not know whether another 'affair' was a good idea now that I and the family were fairly settled.

I arranged to meet Judi on the Friday evening and we had a couple of drinks. We discussed the future and agreed that while we wished to continue seeing each other neither of us should let our developing relationship interfere with my marriage. We saw each other, after that, only when it was possible, asking no demands of each other, and the relationship lasted for over thirteen years until we had a flaming row about monitoring standards of patient care, of all things.

Christmas at the General was very similar to all my previous experiences but this time I was a Consultant and it was expected that the family came to the Unit over the Christmas lunch. The children were thoroughly spoiled and the adults well plied with drinks. There was a turkey to carve for the patients and this was done by Chris.

The RMR Unit also had a very good social life and the highlight of the year was their Christmas Ball. They always, in those days, managed to get a Royal Marine Band and it was so popular that tickets were at a premium. We were encouraged to bring guests from our own walk of civilian life, and people who had helped the Unit in any way during the year.

I invited a GP colleague who had a single-handed practice just round the corner from the hospital and the Unit. His name was Dave Moor and he, as invited, brought his wife. I did not learn till later why there had been a few funny looks from some of those present but he and his wife had split up and he was living with Sylvia, later to be his second wife. His first wife ran the practice and continued to do so until he retired in 1999. Dave, you will recall, was charged, and later acquitted, of murdering a terminally ill patient with diamorphine in 1998.

I was not very impressed with the winter in Newcastle and was longing for some better weather and got the opportunity when a friend of mine in the Navy asked if I would do a locum for him in RNH Stonehouse, in Plymouth, in early March. The whole atmosphere there was more relaxed than in Haslar and I felt much more at home there. The cherry blossom was out in the hospital grounds and it was warm. Several of the colleagues that I had served with in the RN were still in the service as Regulars and it was very nice to see them all again. Several invited me to have a meal with them either in their Wardroom, or their homes. Some of the senior officers asked me to their residences for dinner and to tempt me, unsuccessfully, back to the Navy.

On Otterburn ranges with the RMR the Sergeants were anxious to test my abilities as a Commando trained person. At the end of one session they handed me a rifle and a full magazine. This was a test that, I realised, was in several parts because there is more than simply taking the rifle and firing it. I must have passed the tests as it was all round the Unit the following Tuesday.

I had never thrown a live hand grenade. The 'Doc' is expected to accept any challenge without hesitation. I was a little apprehensive as I had watched the previous thrower, the last of the recruits, throw his such that it went sideways instead of forward and landed in a stream that flowed past the safety barrier. It was a stun grenade and floated on the water past the barrier whereupon everyone threw themselves behind cover as it exploded, giving us all a shower bath. I was relieved when my throw was straight and went off in the right place.

One of my nightmares was unexploded ordnance. In such cases the safety officer has to detonate it with plastic explosive after a safe period of time. The very worst times were when one failed to detonate and so did the plastic explosive charge that Ray Millburn had placed against it. We then had to wait ages before trying again and I could imagine that there would not have been much left of Ray if all three charges had gone off when he was anywhere near. We all heaved a huge sigh of relief when it finally blew up.

It was not possible for me, single-handedly, to provide all the medical cover the unit needed. I asked Hartley if he could second one of the other doctors from the RNR to us at RMR. He agreed to this and sent a newly joined GP from Tynemouth, John Coles. He had no military training but was invaluable as a GP and he gamely tried to get the Green Beret as a Reservist which, for a doctor in practice, is nigh on impossible. He and I got on well for many years.

Muriel, with her triple stables, was beginning to give lessons in dressage to the local teenagers and, eventually, adults. She was very good at dressage and began to compete, and win, in Northern competitions. She very quickly got the BHSAI diploma as she wanted in the long run to be a qualified and accredited teacher.

In July I was to go to a British Association of Surgical Oncology meeting in Nijmegen, in Holland. Muriel and I decided to make it our summer holiday and take the children, who had not been there before.

We thought it a good opportunity for them to meet Auntie Nellie before she got any older.

MoD (Navy) asked for volunteers to be Medical Umpires for a large NATO exercise in southern Norway in mid-September. I put in an application but was shortly after told that Surgeon Captain Cox, Royal Navy, who was our boss on the Surgical Support Team, had decided to go himself.

I thought no more about it until the weekend of the 4/5 September when I answered the phone, at home, to be told by the operator that she had a 'flash' signal for me. This is virtually the highest priority signal in use by the Services. She read it over the phone and it asked me to stand in for Captain Cox who was now not able to go to Norway. I phoned MoD(N) on the Monday saying that I could go in his place on 16 September but that I would need to be back in Newcastle to go to work by 0900 on Monday the 27th. This they accepted as the exercise would have finished by then.

I went down to Plymouth by train on Wednesday the 15th, and we sailed on a cross-Channel roll-on roll-off ferry, about lunchtime the following day, passing up the Channel before turning north into the North Sea. The weather for the first twenty-four hours was good and all the troops enjoyed the food that was laid on by the ship. By the second night it had got very rough and there were only seven of us altogether at dinner that night. I noticed on the ship's licence that she was only allowed to go as far north as Kristiansand, in the summer, and we were heading for Arendal which is just about level with it.

We arrived at first light and started to disembark at 0800. After endless delays we drove to a Norwegian barracks complex where we stayed overnight. The next day it became apparent to me that those in command of things did not realise or accept that I was not part of the RMR contingent who were joining 40 Cdo, or the Surgical Support Team, for the exercise. My notes at this moment read 'altogether chaotic'.

We stayed there until the morning of the 20th when we moved off to set up the BMU (Base Maintainence Unit) for the Commando Brigade, which was made up of 40 Cdo, a Dutch Marine Commando and a Norwegian one. The SST, to which I had by now been unceremoniously attached in spite of my protestations, was to be part of this set-up. When I arrived at the site there was already a real patient needing my attention.

The following day, the 21st, just after lunch a large VW 4*4 Norwegian Army jeep, flying an umpire's flag, arrived in the camp. A very crusty, and obviously annoyed, Norwegian Colonel demanded to know if I was there. He had been trying to find me for two days.

The crusty Colonel who had arrived to collect me was Col. Ivar Johansen from Trondheim. He was a Cavalry Colonel and, when I say Cavalry, I do not mean tanks and armoured cars. He must have been 60, fit as a fiddle and had leathery brown skin. He and his driver sat in the front of the jeep and I shared the back with his radio officer, radios and their rifles. He was obviously suspicious of my military abilities and organisational skills. He was senior to me by three ranks but I was the senior Medical Umpire and could decide exactly what I wanted to do.

On that first afternoon we travelled miles looking at all the Dutch, Norwegian and British medical facilities. At 6 p.m. we went to the Umpires' daily briefing at another barrack complex, at Evjemoor, well to the west of the exercise area. The briefings had started on the 18th, the day we had arrived. I should have gone straight there and my two-day absence had been noted. The Chief Umpire was a Dutch Marine Corps Captain and, when he saw my green beret, I was forgiven. Each section of umpires was expected to give a daily report to the assembled group but I was excused that first night as I had nothing to contribute. It was clear that I would be expected to make up for my absence the following day.

The 'war' had actually started by this time. The Marine Brigade were in the defensive role against an invasion by an American parachute Brigade that had dropped into the area north of us the previous day. It was our job to monitor the battle casualties, killed and wounded being decided by the military umpires, and how they were attended to by the medical services. The most difficult to monitor were the front-line casualties being dealt with by their own first aid, company and unit medical cover.

The Colonel said he would like to visit a Commando HQ in the field. He asked me to take him to see 40 Cdo. No one should be able to find a Cdo HQ as this would mean compromising their position. We set off in the direction of the last known grid reference and turned up a track into the woods, which then began to peter out.

Just as I thought I had got it wrong we almost ran over a sentry who vainly tried to stop us. A few yards further and I only just managed to get the driver to stop before actually driving straight into the Ops tent. I leapt out just in time to meet a furious Martin Garrod, the CO, coming out of the tent, to demand, 'What the f——k are you doing here, Doc?' The appearance of the Colonel calmed Martin down a bit but he was not at all happy that we had found him, though I was fairly chuffed that we had.

I confirmed my suspicions that all was not being played fair with battle casualties and Units were continuing to use all the troops available. At that evening's Umpires' Conference I made the point that in reality the commanders on the ground would not have these troops available. The Chief Umpire instructed all the umpires to enforce this.

The next day we set up a large scale casualty exercise with a simulated air strike on a convoy. We produced 21 'live' casualties requiring finding, first aid, and evacuation from a remote roadside. We were very impressed by the Norwegian Unit's response and they had sorted and moved all the casualties within an hour and a half.

Our SST was in tents and, although there was nothing wrong with its performance, the Colonel and I thought that the facilities were pretty basic and certainly I subsequently always advocated that we set up in a solid building. I was more than delighted when in the Falklands they took over a disused factory.

I was asked to intervene in an amusing episode with 'Prisoners of War'. Our side had captured a number of the American Paratroopers and they had been put on their honour not to escape. They persisted in so doing and the 'Royals' had removed their clothes. The Americans were complaining that they were not being treated correctly according to the Geneva Convention. It was a hilarious sight to see all these naked bodies huddled in the back of a truck. I suggested that if they gave me their word to stop trying to escape I would get the Royals to let them have their clothes back. If they broke their word with me, however, I would personally supervise their removal again. It worked.

Colonel Johansen and I were getting on very well by this stage. His driver took some polaroid photographs of us together and he gave me one as a souvenir. He then reached back into the jeep and produced a bottle of Norwegian Schnapps for me.

The next hurdle was to get home again. I had been told that I was booked on an RAF flight back to Plymouth sometime on Monday 27th. So I caught the 2 p.m. DanAir flight from Kristiansand to Newcastle, on the Sunday, and expected reimbursement of my fare. While awaiting the flight the Brigadier saw me and I explained my situation. He was kind enough to say that if I had any difficulty getting my fare back to let him know.

The flight was in an old BAC 748 twin turboprop. The cabin door was permanently open during the flight and, as both pilots had long blonde hair, it was apparent that both were female. I found this interesting but some of the other passengers were not so generous.

It was time to settle down and begin developing the services for the

Breast Clinic. The Pathologists had just appointed, mainly for the Cervical Screening programme, a new Cytologist called Vinnie Wadheira. She was interested in developing aspiration cytology techniques from solid tumours.

For all the years I had worked in the field of breast cancer I had been totally against the surgical convenience of a frozen section on a biopsy, with immediate mastectomy if it were positive. In a number of ladies we had been able to get a diagnosis of cancer in the outpatient clinic using a Tru-cut biopsy needle under local anaesthetic. The needle was long and large, and it still took a few days to get a result. This new technique used only an ordinary blood test needle and 20ml syringe and an immediate report was possible. Pre-diagnosis allowed time for discussion of the implications of the diagnosis, and the treatment, before any operating was done.

It is most important how the information obtained is used in each individual case. The clinician must weigh the meaning of each result against the clinical and mammographic picture, if available. This came to be known as Triple Assessment and is now the Gold Standard for breast clinics.

Peter Dawes, the Radiotherapist, had brought back to Newcastle a new primary treatment for breast cancer that involved removing the palpable, or major, mass of the tumour and treating the rest of the breast with radiotherapy. This was known as Conservation Therapy, as opposed to Conservative Surgery that, in my view, has always been an inadequate treatment.

In adult solid tumours the cause (Initiator) is mostly unknown, but for about 5 per cent it is genetic. A Promoter helps the malignant process continue once started, and in breast cancer most people believe that it is oestrogens. Removing sources of oestrogens, or preventing them acting with drugs, may stop or slow tumour growth, as certain intracellular enzyme activity is stopped. This does not kill cancer cells but simply stops them dividing or growing, and is called a Chemostatic. This is unlike Chemotherapy which kills cells, both malignant and normal, and is termed Cytocidal.

It should be clear to most people, therefore, that the Initiator and the Promoter may affect all the cells of the target organ, in this case the breast, and – QED – the whole breast requires treatment of one kind or another, be it surgical removal, radiotherapy or drugs.

Until this time all the survival statistics for breast cancer were based on a primary treatment of a total mastectomy in some form. This new Conservation Therapy offered a non-mastectomy alternative. The questions were, in our minds in Newcastle, would it be as good a treatment in the long run and would the ladies actually want it?

In early 1979 we took a decision to discuss the two treatment options with the women once a diagnosis had been made, with cytology, and see if they were able to tell us which they themselves would prefer. The immediate reaction from the female population of Newcastle was not what any of us expected. The women's magazines told us that we were mutilating all these women with mastectomies and there were support groups all round the country to help these 'poor women' get on with life. Everyone expected women to grasp the chance of this alternative treatment with open arms.

In our experience this was not so. The first ten ladies offered the choice were split 7 to 3 in favour of mastectomy. Here was truly a disturbing finding and contrary to popular and professional beliefs and so we published a short paper reporting the finding. It attracted considerable criticism. We approached the Department of Clinical Psychology at the University to see if they would research the issue and so we got the first of several postgraduate students attached to the Unit.

After those first ten ladies the ratio of choice never fell below six to four in favour of mastectomy during the rest of my working life. Our view was that 100 per cent forced Conservation would produce as much, or more, psychological problems as 100 per cent forced mastectomy. In this we were again to be proved right in the long run. We were delighted when our Psychologist supported us.

Surgically I extended the use of aspiration cytology to abnormalities of the liver using laparoscopy, a technique I had also brought with me from Nottingham. This was years before 'keyhole surgery' became a household term. It was galling for me to be told by a rather pompous Senior Registrar, many years later, 'Of course you won't have had any experience of laparoscopy, or colonoscopy for that matter.' I managed to bite my tongue hard.

I went to the British Breast Group meeting in Copenhagen in the spring of 1979. On the overnight ferry home, via Harwich, I was sitting at the bar, minding my own business, when a young woman came and stood beside me. She was blonde and very attractive. She spoke to me in perfect English, although she was Danish, and said that she was having a birthday party on the ferry and would I like to join them at midnight for champagne. Not being a football fan it had all gone totally over my head that she had been George Best's girlfriend.

In March I again went down to Plymouth. The Wardroom in HMS *Drake* was raffling the final sketch for the mural, 'Drake Beating Up

The Channel', by the artist Jim Thompson. I bought two tickets at £1 each. I thought no more about it until I received a phone call telling me that I had won the painting. I have always cherished the painting and it hangs in a place of honour over the sideboard in the dining room. There is a mistake in the painting. Drake is portrayed on the stern castle with a telescope, which had not been invented at that time.

Over the spring school holidays we booked for two weeks in the Saronic Gulf, near Athens. We spent two weeks sailing from village to village, and island to island, visiting Hydra, Spetse and Poros. We had one bad squall. I saw it coming and went to start the engine but for the first and only time on the trip it did not. I radioed my plight to the leader who brought his boat alongside and jumped across. The engine would not start for him either and we were a bit close to cliffs by now. The children were in the cabin looking rather green, and Muriel looking rather white. We decided that we had no alternative except to jibe. In spite of the strong wind I have to say that he and I did a perfect jolt-free jibe and all was well.

The RMR went to Holland with a large contingent from all round the UK. Those from Scotland and Liverpool gathered in our Unit before setting off in convoy to Hull where we took the ferry to Rotterdam and then on to the Dutch Marine base at Den Helder at Doorn, near Utrecht, in the centre of the country.

I was standing at the bottom of a tall Death Slide when one of the young blue berets 'froze' on the platform and refused to go down. A large Dutch Marine Sergeant suggested that I, 'being very experienced', might like to show him how simple it was. This did not have the right effect on the recruit, who refused to budge. Up and down I went several times to no avail until eventually we took his weight off the platform then let go. The Sergeant said in a loud voice, 'Not bad for an oldie.' I was 42 at the time, and it brought home to me that I might be getting just a little too old for this particular role.

These trips were not all hard work and we had a good social life as well. I was roused one morning to be told that our RSM was missing after an evening in the village. There had been no reported arrests or accidents from the local police but there had been a complaint that a bicycle had been stolen. I suggested we check the ditches and gardens and sure enough in the garden of the very last house outside the camp, over the hedge and out of sight of the road, lay the RSM on the grass still astride the stolen (borrowed) bike.

In Utrecht one evening we had a meal and then repaired to a bar in the red light district. The girls, unlike most I have seen in this country, were very attractive, in their late teens and twenties. We felt we had to say that we were not going to be interested in anything except their company. Much to our surprise they said that business was very quiet and that they would be quite happy to stay and be sociable.

I had yet again to return home before the rest. HM Customs decided to be their usual nice selves and made the lads unload all the kit from the trucks onto the quay when they arrived in Hull on the Sunday morning. They said they were looking for drugs. My medical kit, with morphine and pethidine in it, stood unclaimed on the quay throughout, no attempt being made to look inside it.

In the final summer school term we were becoming more and more concerned about Jake's education. We began to consider sending him to a private school, of which there are several in the Newcastle area, but first we sent him to an educational psychologist. He had an IQ of 140, much greater than my own, but was about a year behind any hope of passing the 11 plus exam. He started to have home tuition with a view to letting him try again in 1980.

BASO had accepted our bid to hold the 1980 summer meeting in Newcastle. I, as the local committee member, found myself in the organiser's chair. Joy Gibson, our first conservation choice patient, was a secretary and she agreed to help organise it. This took a load off my mind and once I had booked the University venue and the hotels, I left most of the rest to her.

My concerns about some of Muriel's more dangerous horse activities were confirmed one weekend when she was trying to tame a 'mad' horse. It went wild and she attempted to 'abandon ship'. She went through the fencing of the arena and in the process hit at least one of the fence posts on the way. She ended up breaking one wrist and the opposite humeral neck. She could, of course, do not a thing for herself including taking her pants down to go to the toilet.

My Fiat X/19 was beginning to show the rust very badly and the worst was at the top of the front wings where the shock absorbers were welded directly to the underside. I soon found out that this was their greatest weakness, got it fixed, and traded it in for a new pale green Fiesta 1.1.

A major development, and largely unwelcome, was the opening of Phase 1 of Freeman Hospital, a third large hospital in Newcastle. We four from the General provided emergency cover for Freeman in the anticipation of our eventual move across to the new site in Phase 2. It was extremely inconvenient to be on call for two sites on any one day and night, and involved a lot more travelling. There was, from the earliest days, a sneaking suspicion that Newcastle would end up with three acute general hospitals. This was a very expensive way to provide the required level of service.

The main Accident and Emergency Unit, the Neurosurgical Unit and the Regional Radiotherapy Unit were on the General Hospital site so there seemed to be a certain lunacy about some of the proposals and I determined then to start fighting for the survival of the General as a General Hospital. To some of us it was the ideal combination of a Major Trauma Centre and a Cancer Hospital. It had most, if not all, of the facilities, plenty of room and good communications both within the city, and to the motorway network.

Peter Dawes, I, and the staffs on the two Units, made a Tape-Slide presentation of the two different primary treatments for breast cancer. They were shown it in my office, when I was not present, but the patient could sit with her partner and family, with one of our nurses to help with questions. If, when they had seen the first film, they wanted to see the other one they did and could also see them as often as they liked.

A major headache we had in making the film was in deciding whether to show a real mastectomy scar. It was easy to show the other in the shape of Joy Gibson but we were undecided how the women would react to the full blown 'amputation' scar. In the end we left it in but agreed that we would take it out if there were any adverse comments from the ladies. To assess the impact of this tape presentation a second post graduate psychology student was attached to the Unit.

Little did we realise just how important that single slide was to turn out. What we had failed, as doctors, to realise was that lay people do not know that in a mastectomy the breast (milk gland) is removed from under the skin, the skin put back and sewn together again. The only change in appearance is that that side of the chest is now flat like a man's. The slide convinced those wishing to have a mastectomy that they were not to be left with a round gaping raw area on the chest, which they had thought.

All this was to influence my thinking greatly over the next years as we continued to strive towards greater and greater understanding of the management of these patients. I was also beginning to have great respect for the ability of the 'ordinary woman' to handle information on the subject of breast cancer.

One of our regular visitors, usually on a Wednesday, was Angela Eastwood who would drive up in her plum coloured TR6 with its matching hard top. This made me very jealous especially as it was in immaculate condition. We had heard rumours that she was bisexual and had a girlfriend. Much later, when Angela left Bill to go and live with this girlfriend, Muriel told me Angela had wanted her to be her lesbian partner.

At the General Hospital there was the Regional Medical Physics Unit with Professor Keith Boddy as Head of Department. He had developed whole body scanning to measure people's nutritional state. This scanner, shielded by steel made before the first atomic bomb was exploded, from the German Fleet scuppered in Scapa Flow at the end of the First World War, counts the natural radiation from a person.

My first Senior Registrar, Huw Williams, looked at the nutritional state of patients awaiting oesophagectomy for cancer. We then fed them by a fine bore tube passed into their stomach before, and after, the operation. This did seem to improve their recovery and was a lot cheaper, and much simpler, than intravenous nutrition.

Two other departments in Medical Physics were the Ultrasound Unit, under Tony Whittingham, and the Measurement Unit, under Phil Burns. The former encouraged me to buy a portable ultrasound scanner for use in the clinic to identify cysts, fibroadenomas and some cancers. You can see microcalcification in cancers on ultrasound under certain circumstances, and they can be seen broaching natural tissue planes.

Phil Burns built us patient activated intravenous pumps before there were any on the market. Katie Clarke, my anaesthetist, and I were trying to reduce the amount of post-operative morphine or pethidine that we gave patients as they made them sleepy and not able to breathe deeply when given in the usual way by intramuscular injection. Using the pump we found that only a fraction of the dose was required to get the same level of pain relief.

More significantly no breast surgery, including mastectomy, needed any such drugs post-operatively. The skin incisions do not give the patients the same degree of discomfort as deep trans-muscular ones. Our breast patients could get up and go to the toilet and put their make-up back on, which was a tremendous morale boost to the mastectomy ladies, on the evening of their operation. When I did a mastectomy on one of our own sisters and there was a row when the night sister tried to give her intra-muscular analgesia, those that witnessed it were highly amused.

Jake passed the 11 plus and the entrance exams for King's Tynemouth. We were both very impressed by the school itself and the headmaster, Mr Dillon, in particular. We were pleased when Jake announced that he thought he could be happy there. Fiona was not at all academic and we entered her for Church High in Jesmond. Here the girls were supposed to get a good, all round, education to prepare them for the big world ahead.

Jake got a very rude awakening soon after he started at King's. He was not the tidiest of children and his tie was nearly always loose and his top button undone. He came home one night properly dressed having been accosted by the Headmaster, by name, in the corridor and told to tidy himself up. This image change probably accounted for his decision to stop being called Jake and insisting from then on that his name was James.

In September I got the opportunity to go to Belize, in Central America, to do a locum for the Army. The small garrison was far away from any major surgical facility, the nearest being in Florida. A surgeon and anaesthetist were based there, usually of Registrar grade, to handle any immediate emergencies. The Army was short staffed and someone had volunteered the Reserves to help out.

We flew out from Brize Norton, in civvies, in an RAF VC10 very early in the morning to Washington where the plane refuelled. We were allowed into the Terminal building on our NATO travel warrants and, as the RAF flights are dry, most headed for the bar. We then flew on south over Florida and down the Gulf of Mexico, skirting round Cuba, to Belize. The VC10 was the largest plane to be able to land at Belize International airport and it had to put its wheels down on the black and white markers or it could not stop in the length of the runway.

The time of arrival in Belize was still only lunchtime. There was only the one plane a week from UK, and the person being replaced went back on the same plane so that there would be about two hours to do a hand-over. On this my first trip there I was replacing a RAMC Captain who had just got his Fellowship. He left me a problem in the form of an Army Captain on whom he had done a vasectomy the previous week that had got infected. One of the golden rules of Military Surgery in the 'back of beyond' is that you do not do unnecessary operations.

I had not met my anaesthetist and did not even know if he was on the flight but I caught sight of a Naval white cap sticking out of a bag and assumed that that was his. He turned out to be a Senior Registrar from Harefield's Hospital who spent most of his days doing heart transplants. I wondered how he would find the primitive facilities I envisaged being there.

The military camp is just beside the airport with low, curved, huts tied down with strong wires. The Officers' Mess was mainly atap but the hospital building was also hurricane proof. There was little routine work to be done after going round the patients in the small ward and seeing any new injuries. Once a week the team went up to Belmopan, the new capital of Belize built in the centre of the country.

The new civilian hospital there had a modern operating suite but the air conditioning unit had never worked. The anaesthetic equipment was an original Boyle's machine with small cylinders of nitrous oxide and cyclopropane. The oxygen came from an industrial welding cylinder bolted to the wall and attached to the Boyles machine by thick red rubber tubing. It was so hot that I wore only my underpants, a gown and a pair of surgical gloves.

The cleaner did not mind what time of day she cleaned the theatre, nor if there was an operation in progress. In the middle of a hernia repair the anaesthetic room door was flung open and in she swept, round us, and out through the recovery room door. We just watched, speechless.

The local population were, in general, lovely people who were grateful for anything we did for them. Their only currency was fruit and vegetables and we would return from our trips with bags full from those we had seen and treated. The only hotel in Belize City was the George. We would take a taxi down from the camp and drink in the bar, all the time having to fight off the local girls. Like in all Central and South American countries drugs were in evidence but, in those days at least, there was no trouble.

We were allowed to travel around as much as we like as long as the authorities knew where we were going so that they could send a Puma for us if there was an emergency. I still had a MoD driving licence which allowed me to have a Land Rover so we went off to explore the Mayan pyramids and ruins.

Belize has the world's second longest coral reef and, although not liking swimming, I did go snorkelling. The reef is breathtakingly beautiful and I could just stand on a ledge about three feet wide with a huge drop to the seabed on either side. Two barracudas sniffed my leg and as the boat had drifted away over deep water I had to pull myself together and swim to it. It must be nice to enjoy, and be unafraid of, swimming.

Back home, after this trip, we found that the Georgian house, near Consett, that we had looked at previously was still on the market at a reduced price. We went back and looked at it again although I still had serious doubts. I thought that the fabric of the old building left much to be desired and the outbuildings and stables were somewhat run down. There were 30 acres of land, some woods but mostly grass, which Muriel could see as ideal for training, grazing and perhaps growing crops for feed, hay and straw. I thought that a survey might put her off.

Through James's new school we had met other couples whose sons had also gone there that term. One was the senior surveyor of one of the large estate agents in Newcastle. He did a survey for us and wrote a thick report essentially saying 'not to touch the property with a barge pole'. Muriel was not deterred and as she was going to be putting up a lot of the money, decided that this was what she wanted to start a stable business. We made an even lower offer that was accepted.

Another couple that we met, the Dodds, were very nice and their son, Johnathan, became James's best friend. They owned a small business manufacturing a sort of 'super glue' for bonding wire rope.

We put '159' on the market but the prices had fallen and it looked as if we were going to have a difficult job selling it. This was to turn out to be only too true and we entered the two property situation for the second time. We moved into Priestfield Lodge, as it was called, just outside the village of Burnopfield in mid-December 1980.

CHAPTER SIXTEEN

Priestfield, 1980–1990

P RIESTFIELD LODGE was built in 1862 by a coal baron for his mistress. It was built facing west, not south as is the custom, so that the view was up the Derwent Valley. The road that runs past the house was an old coaching road from Gateshead, across the hills at Whitenstall to Hexham. In the hollow below the house lies one of the coaching stations where they changed horses. The little road is unchanged, very narrow, winding and quite unsuitable for buses and the large number of cars and lorries that use it.

The original house was a typical Georgian square one, four up and four down, with a large hall and a 'low grade' listed staircase with a picture window half way up. A west facing extension had been added on the north side of the house forming part of a courtyard with stables, coach house and hay shed.

The four upstairs quadrants of the house were bedrooms. Leading upstairs from the back door was a very steep staircase for servants to get upstairs without being seen. The staircase went on up to a third floor which had been the maid's bedroom and sitting room. In all there were five toilets, but only three were within the house.

The main drive was down the south side of the house past where a long conservatory had once stood with direct access into the dining room. At the front of the house was a large turning circle overlooking a grass tennis court-sized lawn that, in turn, looked over a hard tennis court and the 30 acres, including the woods, which made up the property.

Muriel felt that this would make an ideal riding business with grazing, crops of hay and wheat (for the straw) and show jumping and cross-country courses. She was intent on setting up such a business although our accountant, myself, and the Inland Revenue were not too sure about the wisdom or viability of such an enterprise.

Within days of us moving in we had a demonstration of the problems in store when in the middle of the night a hot water pipe in the attic burst due to the frost. I clambered up there, nude, with a torch and a wine cork which I pushed into the open pipe and held it in place with a piece of bent Meccano.

There was no mains gas nearer than the village and in an attempt to improve the heating of the house, and at the same time try to reduce the oil fuel bill, we installed a Belgian wood burning stove which was like a poor man's Aga but, theoretically at least, it would burn anything. It was like driving a steam railway engine and given enough wood would easily have equalled Mallard's world speed record. I spent a lot of time gathering and chopping wood every year to feed it.

At first Muriel had only her two horses to look after, and two pupils who partly looked after their own horses on a 'half livery' basis. We acquired our first pieces of agricultural equipment in the form of an old, but large, David Brown tractor and an even older tipping trailer. The manure was put straight into the trailer and dumped by me in one of the fields when full.

Opposite us was Lintz Hall Farm owned by George Tulip who was to become our agricultural adviser and help in the years to come. We first met him, and many of the neighbours, by asking them round at New Year and this established a precedent of renowned New Year's parties over the years. The first one was of modest proportions but later they became quite large affairs.

We registered the family with Dr Ranald McDonald who was in practice in Shotley Bridge. He and his wife Jeannie, who was a part-time Consultant Radiotherapist, became very good friends of ours. They had both trained in Edinburgh and had not lost their strong Scottish accents.

I have always liked to have a local pub that is easy to reach on foot and I was lucky in that the Travellers Rest was at our end of the village. It had a traditional layout with small cosy rooms with fires in them, where the old men of the village would come and play darts or dominoes. Immediately after we arrived the new landlord, Bob, 'modernised' it and made it into virtually one huge bar with a games room at the back.

It was here that I was introduced to a North East tradition – which I knew little about – leek growing. There were fewer than twenty members in our club and we had to pay £1 per week. The main event of the Leek Club, apart from the Autumn Show, was a summer barbecue that was always held at Peter Brown's home in the village. He was the Treasurer of the club. I became the chef for these for several years as I had begun to take a serious interest in cooking due mainly to a need for self-preservation.

I had, by now, got into a routine of getting up early in the mornings with the aid of an alarm clock and a tea-maker in the kitchen, to get the children up and take them into Newcastle to school. They both made their separate ways home. Soon after I met Peter Brown he asked me if I knew that Fiona walked backwards down the hill. She had been seen doing this on her way back from music lessons in Darras Hall. I said simply that it was 'just Fiona'.

I got to the Hospital before 8.30 a.m. and would know what was going on in the wards before the juniors had finished their first round. I could then discuss and solve any outstanding problems with them and the nurses before beginning my day's work. There was adequate staffing to ensure that the work was covered safely and without too much stress to them in terms of on-call commitment.

My workload was increasing, as predicted by Jim Bourke, but I was still thoroughly enjoying it and putting into practice my holistic view of the management of cancer, Surgical Oncology, with the collaboration I had developed with the Radiotherapists, particularly Peter Dawes, Bill Ross and Dick Evans as well as the Oncologists who were given a boost by the establishment of a chair by the University.

The Tuesday multidisciplinary Breast Clinic was expanding fast but not yet at a rate to cause alarm about how to cope. I was still able to see and treat the other interests of mine: peptic ulcer disease, upper and lower gastrointestinal tract cancers and thyroid disease both benign and malignant.

Out of all the thousands of patients I saw there were only four serious litigation attempts against me during my entire medical career. The first, about this time, followed a thyroid operation that was settled after seven years for the cost of a silk scarf to cover the scar of a tracheostomy that someone else had done. The second was a case of a perforated ulcer that was settled after eight years. A third was a lady who developed breast cancer some years after I had seen her, and who had had normal screening mammograms in the interval. She dropped the claim. The last was a rare benign breast condition in which there were two possible lines of action. I realised, in retrospect, that no matter which I chose I would be criticised. This case nearly ended in Court as I defended my decision vigorously until it became clear that 'Catch 22' is only defensible logically. Three of the four were on legal aid.

I could not afford to lose a whole weekend's gardening just because I was on call every fourth week. Muriel could not be relied upon to be there to answer the phone as she would most likely also to be outside with the horses. The solution lay in a radio-phone, now called the cordless phone, but which was illegal in this country. I was able to obtain one from an 'interested' expert. It served me well for many years until they became legal and more numerous, when there started to be cross interference because of the limited number of radio channels.

I learned that the only way I could manage the large garden single-handed was to throw all the seeds into the ground, in rows, over the course of one weekend. Vegetables included cabbages, lettuces, beans (runner, broad and French), beetroot, leeks, cauliflower, broccoli, and brussel sprouts. All I had to do thereafter was to hoe the weeds and thin them appropriately as they grew. With this technique we obtained abundant vegetables most of the year round with minimum exertion.

One of the first priorities was to get Muriel's business started. We increased the number of horseboxes from the original eight to eleven with three new boxes. George Tulip helped us farm the smallholding and in the first year we planted grass and wheat. After this first year we ploughed the hayfield in the autumn and planted winter wheat, and grass in the previous year's wheatfield, trying to achieve a sort of mini crop rotation.

To enable Muriel to teach dressage we converted the hard tennis court to a half sized dressage arena. The old tennis hut in the centre of one of the long sides acted as a spectator base. Later, when we found an old power line that ran down to the hut we became very sophisticated and had a transmitting microphone system to help Muriel teach.

With the increase in number of horses she had to have extra staff. Over the years we had many girls as working pupils; this is a system in the horse world where they are given free riding instruction and tuition, with the aim of obtaining the first of the British Horse Society qualifi-cations, the Assistant Instructor (BHSAI). After some years this was beginning to lose 'political' favour and we found ourselves having to take on YTS (Youth Training Scheme) applicants of both sexes. This was never very successful as there was no real incentive to turn up if they did not feel like it.

The Inland Revenue, not surprisingly, viewed the whole exercise as Muriel's hobby and were very reluctant, certainly at first, to accept it as a serious business. They predicted (accurately as it happened) that there was no way this was ever going to make a profit. They sent a young man down one day to do an inspection. It was raining and although he was obviously supposed to walk round the whole 30 acres and buildings, he only went as far as the end of the lane and declined to go any further into the deepening mud.

One night, after we had been at Priestfield for a few months, Muriel woke up in the middle of the night with severe abdominal pain. I thought this might be a threatened miscarriage. My diagnosis was correct and after all the years we had been married I felt saddened that this was the only chance that we had had to have a child of our own, or so I assumed.

We put Garth to stud and from the resultant litter chose one that had reverted to the French Briard black fur and long tail. He was James's dog and he named him Eccles after one of his favourite Goon Show characters. Eccles ran onto the road, was knocked down and died shortly afterwards. James was inconsolable but we found a Border Collie cross puppy which we christened Eccles 2, although the '2' soon got dropped.

The Victorian swimming pool in front of the house attracted little use except in the very hottest of summer days and after one or two years I gave up the unequal struggle to keep it watertight and the filtration plant working. For many years it was to lie neglected and crumbled further until it was no longer viable as a pool.

We started shopping in bulk at Macro in Washington. Initially we borrowed the Marine Unit's card and one of the Regular staff would have to go with Muriel to do the transaction. Muriel would pay the Marine cash to cover the bill. The very first time this happened she had £100 with her but slightly exceeded this amount and had to borrow from the Marine to cover the gap. I learned through the grapevine, within the Unit, that the Regular staff would have a bet on the size of the bill each time Muriel went shopping.

When the time came to cut the hay we bought a very old hay and straw turning machine. We 'employed' a lad from the village called Colin. He was a lovely, mild mannered, lad who was willing to do anything. Unfortunately he did not know his own strength and tended to break things rather easily but for a number of years we could not have done without him.

The wheat crop itself was taken to George's farm and stored until moved with his own, by lorry, to Piercebridge for storage and eventual sale. This was dependent on the price of wheat at the time. Sometimes we got a good price and sometimes we didn't.

The Navy was still providing Surgical and Anaesthetic cover in Belize for three months a year and I was asked if I would go again in September 1981. I readily accepted and felt like a seasoned visitor. There had been some changes since the previous year as on one occasion the team couldn't be located when needed urgently and this had, not surprisingly, upset the powers that be.

We arrived the day after Independence Day and while the Belize citizens were celebrating our troops were alert for any attempt by Guatemala to take advantage of the situation. There was heightened tension on the border but it led to nothing.

On this visit I did have one real emergency which my own experience helped deal with. A large thunderflash had gone off in a Sergeant's hand. He had been given morphine but when he arrived was still screaming with pain. His hands and face were burnt. He was blind from the flash, like I had been six years previously.

I gave him a large dose of intravenous morphine slowly till he went unconscious. When he awoke I promised him that, based on my experience, he would be able to see again in two days at the most. It worked and he could see again through his still swollen lids within the time scale. He was a very grateful patient.

Well out of my line of duty was cat watching. The wife of the Military Attaché was pregnant with their first child and she had to come down to Belize City Hospital for her ante-natal checks. Her hobby was rearing abandoned baby animals, mainly native to Belize. On my previous visit she had brought down a baby coatimundi, a sort of small ant-eating bear, with a long nose and a very long tongue. I had handled this and it liked to search for ants in ears. It would spend a long time trying in vain, to find one; it was excruciatingly tickly.

She had been brought a cloud leopard cub whose mother had been shot, and who travelled everywhere with her. The leopard was very possessive and protective. As an 'unemployed' officer I was asked if I would look after the leopard while she went to her appointment. The animal looked like a tabby cat but was the size of a large Alsatian. Her canine teeth were fearsome and although she purred like a cat she also had a deep, low, growl for anything she didn't like.

She seemed to like me, I was glad to discover, but there was no doubt that she was in charge. I held on to her rope lead, rather uselessly, while she did what she pleased. They had fed her before coming and she soon became sleepy and yawned with her huge mouth, and not too pleasant a breath. Eventually she decided to go to sleep but, as everyone knows, most cats like to sleep up off the ground so she clambered on to one of the nicely polished officers' mess dining tables.

She lay like any other cat, her huge paws and head dangling over the end of the table, and went to sleep. The Mess Sergeant came and asked me to move her off the table. I suggested he try it himself if he was so keen. He went away, muttering. When her mistress returned from the town she heard the Land Rover arrive, woke suddenly, and took off with a bound in her direction with me trailing behind on the end of the lead.

Auntie Alice arrived at Priestfield, for Christmas and the New Year (Hogmanay) gathering. The house is ideal for these as we could open up the whole of the ground floor for a bar, buffet, dancing and silly games that Muriel insisted on organising. The long hall was ideal for many of the Scottish country dances and I usually could be persuaded to wear my father's kilt for this one occasion a year. One of the girls who kept her horse with us, Jane Riddle, would wear a ridiculously short tartan mini skirt that had all the hot blooded men sweating before they even had one dance. She still wears it today on special occasions, I'm told with the same effect.

It was clear that we would have to invest in a four wheel drive vehicle for the winters. One that had just become available in the UK was the Nissan Patrol. A large 'jeep', it was half the price of the Range Rover and possible slightly larger.

There must have been a certain amount of rebellion in my system during that winter as when I was in London for the Surgical Research Society meeting and the Boat Show, having shaved my chin raw, I decided to grow my beard again. It grew in successfully but it was less red, and more grey, than before. I have never shaved again to this day.

It was thus that we began our second full year at Priestfield and the cycle of gardening and farming went on like that every subsequent year without much change. That year, 1982, was to be different for many people as General Galtieri decided to press Argentina's case for the Falkland Islands by force and invaded them on 2 April.

Following my by now annual routine I did a two-week locum at RNH Plymouth.

Amresh Chakreverty, an orthopaedic surgeon, was due to leave the Navy and go to work in Gibraltar later in the spring. Another friend from RNH Plymouth, the Gynaecologist Dudley Evans, had also recently moved there. Amresh asked if he could come and do a refresher course in General, and other types of emergency, Surgery attached to my Unit. In return I asked that he gave me first refusal for locums out there when he wanted to take a holiday.

We listened with increasing concern when we heard of the raising of the Argentinian flag on the 19th at an old whaling station on South Georgia and predicted that it was only a matter of time before their army arrived to claim the whole island.

One of the first things to happen was that the entire Regular Special Boat Section personnel from our RMR Unit disappeared overnight.

Most, if not all, of my regular Naval Medical colleagues, and other trained staff, found themselves heading south in one ship or another. The manning of the Naval Hospitals was left at a seriously low level and we, in the Reserves, were asked to produce a rota of cover for all the main disciplines.

My colleagues agreed and I went on 15 May, the day after the raid on Pebble Island that indicated to many of us that the re-invasion was very imminent. In the previous two weeks there had been a lot of action off the islands with the sinking of HMS *Sheffield* and the *Belgrano*.

Among the Naval personnel remaining in Plymouth were quite a few on sick leave for one reason or another. I saw a few, in the out-patient clinic, and they were all desperate to join a ship and get involved in the South Atlantic. One case was particularly interesting. A Petty Officer Cook had had an operation on one of his kidneys and was several weeks into convalescence. He was reasonably mobile and pleaded with me to sign him off fit. 'I'm only a cook by trade,' he said.

'Ah yes,' I replied, 'but what is a cook's other job in the event of the ship getting hit?'

His face fell as he realised that I was not as daft as he had hoped. Their 'other' job is in damage control and as a Petty Officer he would be in charge of one damage control party. He simply was not yet ready to return to this 'job' especially after we had all seen, on television, the effects of an Exocet missile on HMS *Sheffield*.

In the middle of my fortnight, on the 21st, the amphibious landing at San Carlos began. We decided to hold a Dining Night for the wives of the doctors from the Plymouth area who were serving in the South.

The dinner was scheduled for 25 May. During the course of the day another of our ships was sunk. We heard that it was HMS *Coventry* but were sworn to secrecy. The wife of their doctor was one of the guests that night. We felt that it was best to continue with the evening so as not to cause any more alarm. Just before the ladies arrived we learned that the doctor had been picked out of the water and was safe: only we were again sworn to secrecy. It was a most ghastly evening with everyone trying to put a brave face on it.

The British Armed Forces, being a volunteer force, ran out of certain highly qualified personnel at an embarrassing time in a conflict. This happened with Helicopter Pilots, Signallers and specialist Medical staff during this crisis. Those who had recently left the service and were still on the Emergency List found themselves called up (most didn't realise this could happen to them) and some, like Amresh, were held beyond their release date.

Any further calling up would have required the Queen to sign individual letters of call-up as the Reserve Forces commitment was 'in the event of actual or apprehended attack on the UK United Kingdom'. Towards the end of the conflict Mr Knott introduced a Bill to Parliament to change this wording.

On 21 June I received a letter from MoD(N) informing me about the 'proposed' changes to call-up. The letter had been written on the 15th and expected a return of a signed proforma within 10 days of that date, otherwise 'I shall assume that there is no serious impediment to your recall.' It transpired that he had had the Order changed back in April even before our re-invasion of the islands.

I replied that I did not feel that I could accept this more stringent, open-ended commitment and I, regretfully, resigned my commission on 12 August. I was later told that the view in MoD was that 'Wilson had got out as he was frightened'. My informant suggested to those assembled that I, in my time, had seen more active service than everyone in the room put together.

I was dined out by the Royal Marines in the autumn, and presented with a large silver salver, thus bringing to an end over 30 years' association with the Senior Service. At 45 years of age I was probably getting too long in the tooth to be with the Royals and I had had an attack of bronchospasm (wheezing) after a recent booster injection of anti-tetanus. The advice from Mike Snow was not to have another one.

I was concerned at leaving the Royals without suitable medical cover. Providence was to take a hand as Ken Queen, from the Nottingham days, applied for a Consultant Surgical post with an interest in Urology at Shotley Bridge Hospital, near Consett, and was appointed. He, like me, was in the RNR, and having congratulated him on getting the consultant job, I told him he had another one lined up at the RMR if he wanted it. I then phoned the Colonel of the Unit and told him I thought I had found him a replacement for me.

Amresh Chakreverty came to Newcastle General Hospital for a month in October/November for his refresher course and then left for his new life in Gibraltar. We again agreed that I would do his locums and so I could foresee that this would replace my RNR and RMR 'holidays'.

While all this was going on Freeman Hospital had opened its General Surgical Wards. To achieve this we at the General were expected to lose one Surgical Ward and the two Consultants, John Chamberlain and Chris Venables. We carefully audited our workload and soon showed that the work was split equally across the three sites and so began to lobby to get our beds restored and replace the Consultant sessions. This proved to be an uphill struggle against resistance from the Health Authority and the RVI. It was to be a skirmish in the continued gradual decline of the General Hospital.

I changed my Fiesta for an ex-demonstration, silver MG Metro. At the end of the spring term we took off in it to France and went south to the Auvergne. At the top of the first pass it started to snow quite heavily, slowing us down so that it began to get dark before we got to the hotel. The MG, being front wheel drive, coped remarkably well and we got there safely.

In May I was invited to go to a meeting in Florence by a drug company for whom I had done some research. It was at the time that the medical profession and drug companies were being criticised for the entertaining that went on. I never accepted invitations that looked as if they were aimed solely at persuading us to use a product. For some obscure reason, maybe because I was giving a paper, I was sat next to the Chairman of the Company, a Lord, at the formal dinner.

James's report at the end of the year was moderately encouraging. He had been doing much better at Tynemouth. Fiona continued to 'enjoy' Church High in her own way which turned out not to be the way her teachers, or the Headmistress, wanted.

Amresh, true to his word, invited me to do a fortnight's locum for him in Gibraltar in the July. The border with Spain was still closed to vehicles, having been shut by Franco in 1966 to vehicles; and completely in 1969. The only way in and out was on foot or by air, or ferry to Morocco. The only flights from UK were three a week by Gibraltar Airways from Gatwick.

To describe the approach and landing at Gibraltar to anyone who has not seen the runway and the surrounding area is almost impossible. The runway crosses the main road that leads to the border with Spain and there are traffic lights to stop the traffic when a plane is landing. Both ends of the runway stick out into the water at either side of the rock and it looks like a very large aircraft carrier.

Similarly it is hard to describe to someone who has never landed on an aircraft carrier what it is like to land in a Boeing 737 at Gibraltar. One approach is straight in over the sea from the east so that the passengers cannot see the runway. The other approach is from the west and as it could not over fly over Algeciras, opposite the end of the runway, the plane flew down the centre of Gibraltar Bay and did a 90 degree right-hand turn at about 1,000 feet above the water, and half a mile from touchdown.

I was accommodated in a hospital flat of St Bernard's hospital. This, like the Naval Hospital a short distance away, is typical British Colonial architecture. There was a second Surgeon, Mr Toomey, simply known to everyone there as 'Toomey'. He was one of the old school of general surgeons who did simply anything that came along. He was ex-Indian Army and treated everyone, including me, as a menial. He was, in spite of his bluff exterior, a hugely funny man with an endless stream of tales of his past career. He was a big man and had a lovely tiny wife who doted on him.

There was not a lot to do in Gibraltar in those days as the economy was fairly run-down. It was sunny and warm, though, and there was a plentiful supply of pubs that sold British beers. I would spend the early evenings in the square with a pint of Courage IPA and the *Daily Telegraph*, on the days that it arrived.

It was possible to walk across the border with Spain through a small gate. No luggage was allowed and I believe it was re-opened really only to let the Spanish workers, who had been employed on the Rock until the border was closed, collect their pensions. Jobs in Gibraltar, previously done by the Spanish, were now being done by Moroccans, who had been brought over specially.

One lunchtime I walked across the border into La Linea and caught the bus up the coast to the fishing village of Estepona about 20 miles away. It was an extremely old bus with barred windows, with no glass in them, full of mainly elderly Spanish with leathered skin. There was a goat on a lead and a few chickens in a basket on someone's knee. It did not take a direct coast road to Estepona but went up several side roads to villages on the way – San Roque, Guardiaro and San Martin.

We passed Sotogrande, famous for its polo and now for the Ryder Cup at Valderama, then along the coast to where they were building a new golf course on the landward side and opposite which I caught sight of some masts. I saw a marina entrance and shouted to the driver to 'stop please'. This he did with some bad grace, I alighted and he drove off. I had no idea where I was or when there was a bus back.

There was a short slope down from the main road at the end of which on the right was a beautiful archway through which I could see the marina. The place is called Puerto de la Duquesa (The Duchess's Port). I fell in love with it instantly and resolved that I would be back. I stayed long enough for a beer and to learn that the bus went to Estepona, where it turned round and that I would be best simply to sit at the side of the road and wait for it.

The other thing to do in spare time there was to sail. The hospital Consultants that sailed had the use of an old Nicholson 32. This was an extremely fast boat that needed a crew of at least three or four to handle safely. Dudley, who had been brought up on Welsh fishing smacks, taught me a lot about the art of sailing on her.

There were of course the Dolphins, far more numerous then than these days; and they would come up the Bay every day looking for food and could be seen daily at about 3 p.m. as they made their way back out again. They are a particularly wonderful sight especially the baby ones. They have a very complicated mating routine and are believed to be the only other mammal that enjoys sex for sex's sake, and they certainly seem to judging by the activity.

Leaving Gibraltar by air is no less exciting than arriving. My first return trip produced an amusing incident as about half way home there was the call from the flight deck, 'Have we a doctor on board?' I always slide down in my seat and hope there is someone else there. At the back of the plane I found one of the stewardesses lying on the floor. Her back had 'gone', she was in severe pain and could not stand. We gave her as much pain relief as we could. I asked her if this had ever happened before. She shook her head and said she was on her first trip after her honeymoon. I couldn't help wondering what she and her husband had got up to.

I had enjoyed my stay on the 'Rock' and returned twice a year for two weeks in the summer and one just before Christmas, every year thereafter until my retirement.

Back in Newcastle we were continuing the fight to keep the General Surgical Unit at the General Hospital. The Health Authority had agreed to replace our Consultant sessions and Malcolm Clague, who had been one of our Senior Registrars, was appointed to share with me. Nigel Jones, a Vascular Surgeon, shared with Alf Petty but spent half his time at Freeman. We did, unfortunately, lose a few beds in the process but were left enough to just be able to cope.

The Breast Clinic was generating a great deal of work now, both out-patient and in-patient. We had introduced a protocol of seeing all patients within two weeks of referral and sooner on receipt of a phone call. This was long before the current National Targets were set in the late 90s. The aim, as with the handful of similar clinics opening in the country, was to get a diagnosis as soon as possible using clinical examination, mammography (plus ultrasound) and cytology. This 'Triple Assessment' technique is now the 'Gold Standard' practice.

Early in the New Year of 1984 ICI invited me to go to Berlin to a conference on Tamoxifen. I was not taken with the thought of Berlin in February, but not wishing to be churlish, asked if they hadn't got anything on somewhere a bit hotter. I felt only slightly embarrassed at asking this since I had done a lot of research for ICI with the drug since it had been ICI 46474.

The reply came back that there was in fact a meeting in Rhodes at the same time and I was welcome to go to this instead if I wished. This meeting was on Wound Infections in Surgery and so I did not feel I would be out of place. It soon became apparent that I was in fact standing out like a sore thumb as there were delegates from all round the world in the field of Wound Infection, and I only knew one of them. I just sat there and tried to look knowledgeable although it was well out of my league.

I was depressed by the content of the meeting in that all the speakers gave papers about the use of prophylactic antibiotics in all the various types of surgery. I have always been against blanket prophylaxis. I could see no need in the majority of cases and I knew enough bacteriology to realise that the bacteria might alter themselves to cope. Only the very last speaker, a Professor from America, echoed my sentiments. He too had been dismayed at the lack of any mention of surgical skill and haemostasis, as major means of preventing wound infections.

It is truly sad that now we are fighting the 'super-bugs' such as Methecillin Resistant Staph Aureus (MRSA) that have largely developed as a result of this prophylactic 'mis-use'. At the General we had strict protocols that were drawn up by Harry Ingham, a bacteriologist. He constantly monitored resistant strains and we had very few. Some of our colleagues in other specialities ignored his policies and had contempt for our efforts at control. We are all paying for this now.

I returned home to find that it had indeed snowed in Berlin and that the unfortunate colleague who had gone there in my place had had to give a paper. I had enjoyed Rhodes so much that I resolved to return for a holiday one day soon.

I was getting tired of the MG Metro as it was too small with the children growing up and it did not have the performance expected of an MG. The same garage had an ex-demonstrator black MG Maestro, a new model, which was only three months old. I bought it and very soon regretted it.

James sat his O-levels that summer and did well, all considering, and got eight. These included English, Maths and Physics and so we decided that he should continue at school with a view to getting A-levels in these and thus a traditional education to get into University to do whatever he decided to do as a career.

He had got to the stage of wanting more money to spend than we gave him in pocket money so that I suggested he got a job for the summer. Our good friend Allan Smith ran Carrick's Bakery in Newcastle and he agreed to put him on the shop floor to learn what 'life' was about. James really enjoyed the experience, learned a great deal and met a lot of interesting personalities.

Towards the end of the summer I received a phone call asking me if I was Surg. Lt-Cdr Wilson by a voice that had the anonymity of the MoD about it. I replied that I was, whereupon the voice asked me to keep the date of 6 November free in my diary, checked my security clearance, and said that I would be contacted again later.

I also received a letter from a drug firm that manufactures one of the first and best known anti ulcer-drugs, asking me if I would go to Baghdad and give a paper at a conference, also in November. They had originally approached one of my colleagues, more versed in peptic ulcer disease, but he had declined in view of the fact that Iran and Iraq were at war and Baghdad was subject to Scud missile attack. I had been suggested because of my military experience (so much for the remarks when I resigned from the RNR). I accepted on condition that I was properly insured for a War Zone (not a cheap option), that I flew first class British Airways and was there as short a time as possible. This in effect meant four days as there were only two flights a week via Amman in Jordan.

The voice of the MoD eventually came back to confirm my availability in Newcastle on 6 November and to tell me that I was required to attend the Civic Centre at 2.30 p.m. dressed in a dark suit. The event in question was the presentation of the Freedom of the City to the 201 General Hospital of the RAMC (Reserves), of whom my anaesthetist Katie Clarke was now the Colonel, by Her Majesty The Queen Mother.

My role was to 'shadow' her medically in case she collapsed. This was highly unlikely as she had more stamina than most of us. I had to carry an airway and a few other bits and pieces secreted about my person, and to be as inconspicuous as possible but within a few feet of her at all times. I was sorry not to have been able to be in uniform but my presence in an aisle seat in about the 3rd row, wearing my Naval tie, in the midst of all the Army uniforms caused not just a little stir. I was asked by several people, some none too politely, what I was doing there?

The Queen Mother was running about half an hour late in a full day's schedule but she left the gathering and crossed the road to where a large number of children were standing and waving flags. Her aides, followed by myself, hurried after her as she departed from the programme, not for the first time that day I guessed, and started to go along the line of children talking to them and accepting small bunches of flowers.

One equerry leant forward and reminded her that they were running very late. The Queen Mother stopped, gave him a withering look and said, 'These children have come to see me so I am going to take a few minutes to talk to them.'

The final part of the ceremony was the march past of the Unit. She took the salute from a small podium with a lone policeman, the only obvious security, standing on either side of it. I hid behind the podium and moved from one side to the other so that I had a clear view of Her Majesty. There were only the four of us on that side of the road. After the parade had passed she turned round and smiled at me as if to say 'thank you'. I am sure that anyone who has been lucky enough to receive one of her smiles will never forget it the rest of their lives.

The trip to Baghdad was two weeks later. I flew out on Sunday 18 November to return the following Wednesday. I had had to apply for a visa and I had been briefed on some dos and don'ts in Iraq. The British Airways Tristar flew to Amman, where it refuelled, then on at low level, in the dark, across the desert to Baghdad. We arrived at 15 minutes past midnight. It was very hot and we arrived just behind another plane carrying about 200 immigrant workers. The queues for the immigration were huge. It was clear that it would be a long wait.

I stopped a security guard and tried to explain the problem. He gave me a glare and went off. He returned a few minutes later and took me firmly by the arm, pulling me out of the queue and inserting me at number two. At about 3 a.m. we got into a minibus and drove, through the red traffic lights, into Baghdad and the Meridian Hotel.

I had the next day to myself and went for a walk. Just round the corner from the hotel was a street that was Baghdad's 'Harley Street'. Signs advertised all forms of Medicine and Surgery. There was one that read 'Varicose Vein, Haemorrhoid and Hernia Surgery' then an Arabic name with the letters FRCS (Ed) (Failed).

I then crossed the new, wide Al Jamhoriyah Bridge. Half way across the bridge was an elderly Arab sweeping the pavement with a broom. He stopped to let me pass. At the end of the bridge I turned left into what was obviously an Arab quarter. I was beginning to wonder if I was safe on my own when I came across some small boys playing football. The ball came in my direction so I kicked it back and then played very bad football for some time.

The elderly Arab was still there as I re-crossed the bridge. On this occasion our eyes met. He put the broom down and placing his hands together bowed deeply saying something in Arabic. I returned the gesture and knowing no Arabic simply said, '*Effendi.*' He gave me a huge toothless grin and proceeded to chatter away in Arabic. We had a long, wide ranging conversation about the weather, the river and the fact that there were few fish in it these days, the traffic volume on the bridge, how it took him nearly all day to sweep both pavements and, somehow, that I was a doctor. In the end we repeated the greeting and the deep bows.

The Peptic Ulcer session was one of the first so I was looking forward to getting it over with. I sat on the end of the first row waiting to climb on to the rostrum and was amazed to hear the chairman announce that there was no need for me to give my paper as Iraq couldn't afford H2 antagonists and that there were cheaper and simpler options, including eating Egyptian Cabbage.

The representative and I were shaken at this and I thought 'whoops', they have just spent £2,500 for nothing. That night we went across the street to the Sheraton Hotel for dinner. We had the attention of two very pretty Philippine waitresses. As we were leaving, and the representative paid the bill, they asked for our room numbers. He wrote something on the back of his 'card' and we left.

At 6 a.m. there was loud knocking and before I could get out of bed the door burst open and two men and the manager burst in. They rushed round the room looking everywhere including in the wardrobe and under the bed. I demanded to know who they were and what they were doing. They announced that they were the Religious and Moral Police, and had been informed that I had a girl in my room. They were clearly annoyed to have had a fruitless search and they left with extreme bad grace.

The next day three of us decided to visit Babylon. One of the representatives hired a taxi and the official guide who had to accompany all visitors. Very little of the buildings were still visible in Babylon, and only the outline of the layout could be seen in the sand. There were a few decorations on them but these were not the ornate ones I expected. Most interesting was the meeting of the river Euphrates with the sand and the rushes. As portrayed in the Bible the three merge imperceptibly into one another and it is easy to step from sand and rushes into water in a single pace without realising it except the shoes get wet.

Back in Baghdad I went off on my own again to the Souk. Here they sold everything and if they didn't have it they made it from scratch. I felt perfectly safe with the locals and they were all very friendly.

The process of leaving Iraq was just about as long and complicated as when I arrived but I had learned to call myself Ronald, not Wilson, as they file by our Christian name and it was a great relief to us all to get on the plane.

I think it was during this trip that Garth died from a heart attack. We eventually found a replacement, male Old English and named him Joe. He was smaller than Garth and as thick as two short planks. He spent a lot of his days chasing aeroplanes off the land. He was very pleased with himself as they didn't come back.

It was becoming clear that James was not doing well in his first 6th form year. One contributory factor to the change in his performance was the loss of the headmaster, Mr Dillon. At the end of the summer term we had a parents' night at James's school and were advised that perhaps we should not waste our money and their time, and James's, keeping him there another year. We were very depressed towards the end of the evening and only had the Art teacher left to see.

She looked at us earnestly and announced, 'James has got talent, you know.' We were speechless as we had never taken any notice of, or interest in, his artwork. She assured us that this was correct and in view of his poor performances in the main subjects suggested that we should consider sending him to North Tyneside College of Further Education to do an Art course.

The last member of the Gordons, the older Aberdeen generation, Auntie Alice, died in April 1985. The estate had to be wound up and No. 9 put on the market. The oil boom of the 70s had stopped and we had considerable difficulty in selling it. It lay empty for a time and as a result some weather damage occurred before a buyer was eventually found. It has now become a Casino.

Muriel needed a full size dressage arena, so we extended the original 'tennis court' again. To get a base that would allow an eventual continuous surface required hundreds of tons of masonry rubble, covered by sand, rolled and compacted. I did this last job myself driving a large hired vibrating roller up and down for seemingly ages. In the end I took to reading a book rested on the handlebars.

A frequent visitor to Priestfield was a dressage instructor called Danny Pevsner. He was an Austrian, of Israeli extraction, and certainly the most grumpy and boorish man that I have ever met. He came up to Priestfield once a month to teach Muriel and some of her pupils. He was a Fellow of the British Horse Society of whom there are only a handful at any one time. Danny believed that one day Muriel would be invited to sit the Fellowship. In the meantime both she and her best pupils began to win more and more Regional and National Dressage competitions.

In September we hosted the meeting of the British Society of Gastro-enterology in Newcastle. Chris Venables' reputation as a gastroenterologist was widespread and he had also been known to do gastroscopy in animals.

One day his phone rang and was answered by his daughter. The voice at the other end announced that he was the King of Spain's vet. Not surprisingly she put the phone down.

The caller came back and it *was* the King of Spain's vet. They had a sick panda. Chris went to Madrid and gastroscoped the panda who had severe gastritis. He prescribed an H2 antagonist and a diet of milk chocolate to replace his normal bamboo shoots and it recovered.

At the beginning of the University year James started Art training. He had passed his driving test first time and as the College is a little off the beaten track I bought him an old red Ford Fiesta. This was to serve him, and later Fiona, as a trusty steed for some years.

The year 1986 was to see some radical changes in my life both professionally and personally. Professor Forrest produced his famous report on the feasibility of population screening for breast cancer in the UK. Mrs Thatcher, who was facing a General Election, immediately accepted the report and instructed the Department of Health to put it in place.

Our Combined Breast Clinic, and the Cancer facilities at the General was an ideal base upon which to establish a service to serve the north-east part of the Region and as a pupil of Professor Forrest I was excited at the prospect. It was not to be as simple as that as I had not made allowances for local medical politics and my deteriorating relationship with the Professor of Surgery.

At this time I was nominated, by my colleagues through the local committee, for a 'C' merit award. I immediately decided to get rid of the awful Mark I MG Maestro and changed it for the new Mark II version. It had a very annoying computer voice that kept telling you what you were doing wrong but it was a very nice car to drive.

I had grown fond of Gibraltar itself and had fallen in love with Andalucían Spain, and Duquesa in particular. I went to work there again in the July and took the whole family with me for the first time. The children, like me, loved it but Muriel, always wanting to be on the go, found it boring and not really to her taste.

With the opening of the border the economy had started to get better and work had started on building some new apartment blocks at the side of Shepherd's Marina called 'The Water Gardens'. I felt that I was going to have a long term attachment to the 'Rock' and wanted to invest in one of the top floor apartments in the first block. The price was £20,000 for a two-bedroomed one with a good view over the Bay.

Muriel, unfortunately, was not at all interested and would not agree to it. Having had this plan rejected I quickly went to plan 'B' and said in that case I would buy a boat.

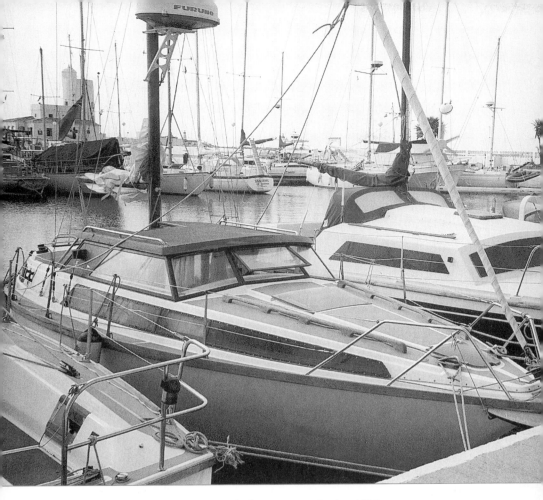

Murella in Puerto de la Duquesa, Spain, 1986.

The Eye Surgeon, Jan Brass (a Belgian), had moved his boat from Gibraltar to Duquesa and he suggested that I look up there, or at Estepona, for a boat. The next time I was in Gibraltar I hired a car in La Linea and drove up for the first time on my own.

I was looking for a reasonable sized boat that I could sail single-handed but that had good accommodation. In Estepona I found just such a boat, a Fjord 28 motor sailer. The first time I saw the boat she was out of the water for a hull clean and a coat of anti-fouling. She also had a very long and heavy keel, needed for good stability and safety. Her name was *Murella*, which means 'walled garden' in Spanish. How they came to call her that I do not know but she had a cruiser stern with very high coaming, a good safety feature, for rough following seas off Norway. She was fully registered and had a 'blue book' that acted as a sort of passport and was more valuable than a small ship's registration.

I bought her and she cost about half what I had wanted to spend on the apartment in Gibraltar. While probably not as comfortable she had four permanent berths and two more occasional ones, a shower (cold) and a small but neat galley with a cooker and fridge. I decided to take her to Shepherd's in Gibraltar but first I had to go back to nautical school and relearn some skills, and learn some I had not done before. The most important new skill was to get my radio operator's licence that required I did a course at South Shields.

James had done really well at College and got 'A' levels in Geography and English Literature as well as 'O' levels in his newly chosen subject of Art. He decided to stay there and embarked on a two year course to get 'A' levels in the art subjects with the aim of eventually getting to University by this rather roundabout route.

In the spring I wanted to show Muriel the boat but she was not too keen because the living was a bit Spartan although there was a shower bloc in the Marina that was basic in the extreme. She wanted to get out and about, and so we hired a car and went through the mountains, and the National Park, up to Jerez. This is where the sherry comes from and where the Spanish Riding School is based. Muriel went to watch them training and I repaired to a tiny bar just round the corner. The old Spanish men were drinking chilled Fino sherry and chilled Rioja at 10 a.m.

Back home there were moves afoot at both the District and the Regional Health Authorities as to how to implement the breast screening programme. Determined to be involved I wrote to Professor Donaldson, the Regional Medical Officer. He wrote back inviting me to become involved in the working party to develop the service. At District level I was not so welcome as the fight for control within Newcastle had already begun. The Health Authority wanted to put the Newcastle Unit at NGH but there was stiff resistance from the Professor.

In April I moved the boat to Gibraltar. On this first trip I was lucky and it was a very smooth trip. It takes about five hours to Europa Point and provided it is an easy passage round the corner it is about another hour to Shepherd's Marina where I was allocated a berth well into the marina and third in from the end of the pontoon. This was her home for the next five years.

James wanted to go out and live on the boat for the summer. I said that I would pay the airfare but that he would have to get a job. He got one painting boats in the marina and as he had shown himself to be a good handyman was in demand. I had put him in touch with Dudley but unfortunately he and David, Dudley's son, did not hit it off. He did make friends with the son of the sailmakers Jim and Jan who lived on the boat opposite. He organised to go back the following year and was much more confident that he would get employment.

At a Christmas party given by Charlie and Janet Thompson, one of my anaesthetists, I experienced severe chest pain. I did not have any other symptoms and I did not collapse. It persisted for some time so I got Muriel to take me home. By the time I got home the pain had gone. Ranald came to see me and arranged a domiciliary visit by a cardiologist who could find nothing wrong either, and my ECG was normal.

I then began to have attacks of bronchospasm with severe wheezing and difficulty in getting my breath. In all I had three severe attacks over the next eighteen months. They were all associated with the consumption of dry white wine. I did some reading and found that in Germany a number of people had been very ill from drinking white wine that had been made drier by the addition of sulphites. The wine industry said it was a lot of rubbish but I decided to take no chances, as at least one person had died from it, and stopped drinking all but the most expensive and well-known brands.

It was apparent to me that if we were to be the Centre that assessed screen detected abnormalities, and I was to become the Programme Manager, we were going to need more staff. I could not handle any more on my own and I would need a colleague to cover when I was away and vice versa. The DGM agreed to this and following shortly afterwards Clive Griffiths, also from Nottingham, was appointed.

John Farndon went to Bristol to be the Professor but, unfortunately, the Professor announced that the Breast Clinic would continue at the RVI to be run by John's replacement. It was a great pity that all of the breast work could not have been centred at the General. I always have felt that this was a missed opportunity. He also made yet another attempt to get the screening based at the RVI. At a very difficult meeting in my room at the General, with Dr Pledger of the DHA, I just had to say NO to the Professor, and spelt it for him, 'NO'.

In April we got the funding through for the Screening Unit. We planned to static screen and assess at NGH, and have two mobile screening vans to tour the rest of the area we were to screen once every three years.

James and Fiona flew out to Gibraltar at the end of the summer term. Fiona had been going to Derwentside College to do a Secretarial course. She had been learning shorthand, as well as typing, and I was confident that she would get a job fairly quickly. Indeed she began work the afternoon after she arrived as the temporary PA to the Manager of the Rock Hotel as there was hardly anyone there who could do the job.

James was joined in Gibraltar by his friend Johnathan while I flew out for five days towards the end of their holiday. The four of us set sail to go up the coast to Duquesa. As we crossed the end of the runway on the east side of the Rock a huge gust of wind down the runway blew us over. I thought for a moment that we were going to take water over the side but the high gunwales and the sheer weight of the keel saved us as I let go everything and we bobbed up again like a cork.

We got to Duquesa without further trouble. In the morning Fiona pointed out that she was due to fly back to UK that lunchtime, a fact that had completely escaped my attention. James, Fiona and I piled into a taxi and raced back to Gib. The following day we sailed back to Gibraltar but Johnathan decided he had had enough of sailing and decided to take the bus. James and I got back without incident.

In the Breast Clinic we had employed another post graduate psychology student to look further at the issue of choice of primary treatment and how women reacted to the offer of choice. She confirmed women could handle the choice, given sufficient information. One of the frequent comments by the patients was that it was most unusual for the patient to be asked her opinion. The ratio of mastectomy to conservation remained at 60/40 and there was no difference by age, menopausal status, social class or any other parameters we looked at. It was simply a personal preference.

After 150 patients had chosen we submitted a paper to the *British Medical Journal* in the autumn and it was published in the November. It created a further storm of criticism but we were delighted when it eventually became accepted practice across the United Kingdom, although the actual methods used varied from Centre to Centre.

James had done very well at North Tyneside College of Further Education and came out with sufficient qualifications to realise his ambition of going to a Scottish University. He started at the Duncan Jordonstone College of Art in Dundee and for the first year he elected to live in college. He was a bit miffed when, after all his work to get there, he was nicknamed 'The Englishman'. Fiona completed her secretarial course and got a job in the works department of the General Hospital.

That same month we began the detailed planning of the Screening and Assessment Unit to be housed at the General. We had to find staff and employ them to run this service. This was easier said than done as there was a shortage of radiographers and, even more so, of radiologists with screening experience. We were very lucky in that the Department of Plastic Surgery attracted an application from Neil McLean whose wife Lesley was just the person we needed to run the Radiology side of screening.

We were equally lucky to get Carol Mallen as the Screening Office Manager, Sue Park as the Superintendent Radiographer and Sandra Horsefield as the Macmillan Breast Care Nurse. These four initial appointments were still in the Unit throughout the rest of my clinical job and indeed Lesley took over from me as Programme Manager.

Just before Christmas I was struck by another attack of severe central chest pain. Although it had gone by the time I got to the General I spent the night in the Coronary Care Unit but again all the tests were normal. I wondered if there was a connection between the breathless attacks and the chest pain. Within a few weeks we had established that I was suffering from an allergic reaction. White wine and some perfumes were my main problem. I started to carry an inhaler at all times. I was naturally pleased that there was not a cardiac cause.

I was invited to be an examiner for the College in Edinburgh for the final Fellowship exam. It certainly kept one on one's toes, and up to date with surgical practice.

It had been a concern of mine since I saw the plans for the National Screening programme that the proposed method of evaluation of the success or otherwise of the programme was to be based only on time to death. There were many surgical and medical treatment options available singly and in combination, primary, adjuvant and subsequent. I believed that poor or inadequate treatment might undermine the chances of screening improving not only survival, but the quality of life, by preventing recurrence. I was certain that the treatments used on an individual required monitoring.

In some trepidation I approached the National Co-ordinator, Muir Grey, and floated the idea to him. To my surprise I was invited to the DOH to put my case. After discussion with the computer team they agreed in principle to develop a treatment recording system as I had suggested. I was allocated money to develop a system into one that would be acceptable to my clinical colleagues. The Screening programme would develop a module to be able to transfer data electronically between the two.

I was asked by Muir to be the Surgeon on a committee reviewing the Assessment process and documentation. The document 'Organising Assessment' was published the following year. At the time there was no other Surgeon showing interest in what I felt was a vital part of the screening chain and became a member of the National Evaluation Group which was going to have to look at the long-term benefits, or otherwise, of the programme over at least a ten year span. These decisions threw me into a new set of national meetings requiring frequent trips to London. All this was leading in the direction of Quality Assurance systems for the programme.

I decided to do a short course in General Management and went to Aston University in Birmingham for a few days. I was pleased that many of their ideas coincided with my concept of management that I had been used to in the Navy and which was different from the management style that was creeping into the Health Service.

On the home front I decided that the old swimming pool was becoming an eyesore and decided to turn it into a large pond. To do this I hired a half-sized JCB and drove it into the middle of the pool and used the bucket to pull the edges towards the middle and slope them inwards. The two dogs thought that it had been built for their enjoyment and nothing would stop them going in swimming.

I could no longer read the telephone directory easily and asked Roger Gillie to test my eyes. He soon found that I needed reading glasses but to our horror my ocular pressures were well above acceptable levels. He prescribed some eye drops to try to reduce it.

In May we opened the Screening and Assessment Unit at the General. It was apparent that Clive and I would need still further clinical help. We were lucky to be able to appoint Angela Brady as our Clinical Assistant that meant that we had a female member of the clinical team on a permanent basis.

On 12 July we had the official opening ceremony performed by Diana Moran (the Green Goddess), the physical fitness expert. She had had bilateral mastectomies the previous year and had just written a book about her experiences. She had just got married and had delayed her honeymoon to open our unit.

In the September we were saddened to hear that Uncle Jo Wondergem had died. Had my father lived he would have been 83 although I think Jo would have been slightly older. I was sorry not to have seen him more in the latter years.

In the October I received a letter informing me that I had been elected to the prestigious Moynihan Chirurgical Club. This is a travelling club for Surgeons and their wives from Teaching Hospitals outside London. John Chamberlain had asked if I would like to be considered for membership as Peter Dickinson was retiring. Muriel and I were invited to the next meeting in Oslo the following May.

James, who had joined the RNR in Dundee and taken over my uniforms, went down to Dartmouth for his Commissioning Course. I briefed him as best I could as to the likely pitfalls and was pleased that some of my tips had proved correct and useful. He passed, which did a lot for his self confidence. Fiona had inherited the Ford Fiesta from James but it had been stolen and found burnt out in the West End of Newcastle. It was a sad loss after so many years and as she was now without transport I bought her a 'nearly new' Fiat Panda for her birthday.

British Leyland had just announced that they were going to produce a special edition MG Maestro Turbo with bodywork by Tickfords. Only about 300 of them were built to order. I took delivery of a British Racing Green one and, once mastered, it handled wonderfully. It was the most powerful production saloon car at the time.

Muriel, as predicted, had been asked to apply to sit the Fellowship. She worked very hard for it, there being a lot of theory to brush up on. Like the Surgical exams the candidates have to pass all parts, or at least specified parts, of the exam at the one and the same time. This makes it even more difficult to obtain the qualification and indeed Muriel failed on one of the vital parts when she first sat it. We were all optimistic that she would pass it one day.

There were two further developments in the Screening Programme. The first was a local initiative by the local morning paper, the *Journal*, to collect money so that we could offer screening to younger women with a family history. One of the ideas for fund-raising was to hold literary lunches. In November we had Simon Weston, the authors Daniel Easterman and Dorothy Dunnett, and the publisher Liz Calder. The second was a National initiative to study the optimum interval between screens and we were asked to participate.

At the beginning of December 1989 I saw Roger Gillie again and depressingly found that the pressure, which had initially fallen with the drops, had risen again. He suggested trying a Beta-Blocker in drop form as although I was an asthmatic only 5 per cent of patients absorb enough from the eye to exhibit side effects. We were both relieved that the pressure fell again and we had high hopes that it would be maintained this time.

Early in the New Year we noticed that Eccles was limping and then started not to use one of his hind legs. An X-ray revealed that he had a tumour (sarcoma) of his acetabulum (pelvis/hip socket). Dogs can function on three legs and he had an amputation. He had no problem on three once he realised that he could no longer lift a leg against a tree.

Our optimism about controlling my ocular pressure with Timoptol was short lived as I began to get side-effects from absorbing the drug from the eyes. I began to have hypotensive episodes, and nearly fainting. My pulse rate had dropped from its normal 60 a minute, since the Royal Marines, to 42. Roger, reluctantly, suggested that I would have to have bilateral trabeculectomies where a new opening is made into the eyeball under the upper eyelid.

It was not an operation that was done routinely in 1990 for pressure changes only in a relatively young patient with a job as a Surgeon. Roger said that he would do the two eyes separately, a month apart. I immediately, and correctly, interpreted this to indicate a risk of blindness resulting if the operation went wrong.

I was admitted to Walkergate Hospital and the first operation was done the next morning. I had never had a general anaesthetic before and was petrified. Rob Bullock gave the anaesthetic. One of my first visitors, after the family, was Ken Queen who presented me with a toy parrot to put on my shoulder. Roger agreed to do the second side the following week. It also went extremely smoothly and I got home very quickly indeed and went back to work in early June.

Although only a few weeks after the operations, Muriel and I went to our first Moynihan Club meeting in Oslo in the middle of May. This was a truly new experience as it is a mixture of science and socialising with the hosts and downright good fun when the club is on its own.

James and Fiona were still interested in learning more about sailing so they went together to the north west of Scotland where they did the Coastal Skipper's course. They both passed all the parts of the test but poor Fiona failed to get enough sea hours experience in, because of bad weather, and so did not get the actual certificate.

It became apparent that Eccles's tumour was recurring and although he struggled on it was clear that he was suffering more and more pain so reluctantly we had to take the difficult and sad decision to have him put to sleep.

Muriel wanted to build an indoor arena so that she did not have to stand outside in the winter to teach. The building was to double as a hayshed and was designed like one. The builders assured us that it was quite acceptable as an agricultural building and did not need planning permission as we already ran a smallholding. This was to prove incorrect due to the size of the building and retrospective planning permission had eventually to be obtained.

Muriel was also judging Dressage events in other parts of the country as well as competing in them herself at National level. For some of the longer trips to the south she borrowed my MG. I had wanted another Jaguar and found a manual 3.4L Cabriolet. It was a lovely, if rather expensive, car to drive especially with the hood down but useless in snow.

The new extension to the screening unit, for the two additional studies, was finished in the late autumn and we asked Diana Moran back again to open it. This time she asked to visit the ward and meet some of my patients. It so happened that there were five ladies who had undergone mastectomy that week. When we got to the ward none of them were to be seen but as it was a beautifully sunny November day we found them all sitting outside.

Spain had joined the EU and I moved *Murella* up to Duquesa so that she would be in a more sheltered mooring over the winter. I was very lucky in that I got berth 272 which is in the centre of the marina and facing east. To get this cost me four bottles of wine.

Soon after I returned I came home from work one evening to find that our old friend from the Bristol days, John Allan, had turned up feeling sorry for himself as his second wife had just left him for a younger man. His first wife had died of breast cancer and his second had been one of the nurses who had looked after her. He stayed for a long weekend, and we did our best to cheer him up.

The year came to a close marking our first ten full years at Priestfield. I felt that I was probably at the peak of my professional career but most of my salary was going on the upkeep of the place that was undoubtedly crumbling faster than we could afford to prop it up. Our 'friend' the surveyor had been undoubtedly correct to advise against purchasing it. My only 'spending money' came from my 13th month salary from my locums in Gibraltar that had virtually become my second home.

CHAPTER SEVENTEEN

1991: *Annus Horribilis?*

T HE YEAR 1991 started, as most of the recent previous years had, with me sitting on the David Brown '95' tractor while emptying the muck trailer twice a week; on a Wednesday, after work in the dark, and at the weekend often in the freezing wind or driving snow, working out in my head how many more trips I would be doing until the spring and I could get into the garden and greenhouse again.

I was at the peak of my career in terms of achievements but finding that the part-time handyman's job was wearing me down. Priestfield was taking an enormous amount of upkeep to stop it actually falling down and a fortune to keep even remotely warm in the winter with the oil-fired central heating.

It was an awakening event, therefore, to come home one dark evening after a 'hard day at the office' to become aware that Muriel had been having sex with someone. Our arrangement on extra-marital affairs still stood and I mused over who it might be. A few weeks later I came home, in the dark, to find that Muriel was not at home. She returned shortly after and I again realised that she had recently had sex.

I now decided the time had come to find out what was going on. I realised that since I had bought the Jaguar Muriel was borrowing the MG regularly at weekends to go off on courses, competitions and teaching trips, mainly down south. I wondered if there was a connection between these increasingly frequent trips and her sexual activity.

I employed the old radio intercept technique to try to find out if I could identify a place that she could visit as part of these 'horsy' trips, but that was separate from them. I got a map of the south of England and began to plot on it all the places she had been to over the autumn and winter months, and drew lines between those places diagonally opposite each other. To my surprise this produced a small central box in the middle of which lay the town of Swindon where John Allan lived.

In the light of our longstanding agreement about affairs, and my own extra-marital relationships, I was not really in a position to say, or do, very much as their relationship had not impinged on our marriage. This situation was not to last very much longer. John, a great caravaner, hired a caravan in the park on the bank of the Tyne at Hexham where Muriel met him.

One weekend I noticed a sheaf of letters. Curious, I looked at the top one and in capital letters was the word LOVE several times. They were from John to Muriel. From them it was clear that there was more to their relationship than just a fling and one contained the comment: 'Poor Ron – when are you going to tell him?'

This I was not prepared to accept and determined to start taking steps to protect myself and my interests. From the Yellow Pages I selected a lawyer specialising in 'matrimonial problems' and went to seek his advice. He was very helpful and having listened to my story shook me by telling me that I had only a short time to confront Muriel with my knowledge as, in law, if I delayed beyond three months I was seen to be accepting the situation. I would then not qualify for a quick divorce. In addition I would require more concrete proof of infidelity than I had at present to convince a court should it come to that.

I set about obtaining more evidence. I cannot say that I enjoyed getting into the realms of sleuthing but as the evidence came in it was clear that this relationship was more than a simple fling. Armed with the additional evidence I went back to David who felt that this was sufficient for the court.

After a lot of thought, and with trepidation at stepping into the unknown, I sat her down one evening just before Easter 1991 and told her that I knew about her and John. She was clearly taken aback but did not deny it. She did, however, after getting over the initial shock ask questions obviously aimed at determining how much I knew.

After some time and discussion she admitted that they had fallen in love and wanted each other. I replied that she would, in that case, have to choose between him and me as I wasn't prepared to share her affections. It took her less than an hour to decide that she would prefer to be with him and this speedy decision confirmed my view that I had only just pre-empted the reverse confrontation. Further confirmation came soon after when, having phoned John, she announced that she would be leaving at the end of June and taking all her belongings in the horsebox.

James and Fiona had to be told. I said that in the light of the circumstances I felt that it was up to her to tell them and explain herself.

She told Fiona when she got home from College and phoned James in Dundee later that evening. They were both, of course, devastated.

I moved into one of our spare rooms at the opposite end of the house. My passport was somewhere in the postal system getting a USA visa put in it so that I could not even escape to the boat in Spain. Instead I took off to Jersey over the Easter weekend.

I did not tell anyone at work about our separation and decided not to until after the trip to Canada. I had had to tell the Club Secretary that I would be coming on my own but did not say why. The only people in the group I told were John and Mary Chamberlain. Some of our other close friends tried to broker a reconciliation but I knew that there was no chance of that happening in the light of my understanding of their relationship and their plans.

It was the 40th birthday of one of our Staff Nurses in the middle of May, just before I went to Canada. Her name was Sue Sewell and she had joined the Unit in 1989. I decided, being unattached, to join them for a drink at their first pub. She was married with two children but I found that I could talk to her easily. At the two previous Christmas nights out I had danced with her and given her a goodnight 'peck'. I must have been feeling very brave, lonely or tipsy, as I asked her if she would meet me for a drink when I got back from Canada.

The Canada trip occupied the first half of May. I was somewhat depressed but the trip started on a light-hearted note as I arrived alone, when booked as a couple, and Michael Wilson, my old boss from Bristol, arrived with his new wife, Marjory. All the hotels got the rooms, and the luggage, confused between the two Wilsons.

I shall be eternally grateful to John and Mary Chamberlain, and other members of the Club, who were very sympathetic and supportive once they had been made aware of the situation. The Club has its serious moments in surgical science, but it lets its hair down frequently and easily. On the dot of noon on the bus, in the middle of the prairies, between Edmonton and Calgary, the gin bottle appeared accompanied by plastic cups, tonic and ice. There was beer for the rest of us.

Those of us that were staying a second week travelled on a Brewster's tour from Calgary to Vancouver, via Banff. We went up Sulphur Mountain the base of which is at just over 5000ft on a cable car to the top at 7500ft. I loathe cable cars and was nursed to the top by Ena and Colin Davidson. The next day we drove up the Icefields Pathway, visiting Lake Louise on the way to the Athabasca glacier.

We then set off westwards through the Rockies to Kamloops, where we stayed the night at the Lac Le Jeune Resort. The lake there had just unfrozen and I hired a canoe. I set off up to the other end of the lake but had difficulty getting back due to the wind. On the final day we followed the Fraser River down to Vancouver.

The time I had been able to spend alone on the trip had given me ample opportunity to think about the future. By the time I returned home I was much more settled and determined that I would take control of the situation regarding a divorce and division of the assets. It was not an easy homecoming as I told Muriel that I was filing for a 'quickie' divorce on the grounds of her adultery. She accepted this but asked me not to name John. I was speechless.

Among the large pile of mail awaiting my return were two letters that lifted my spirits and made me chuckle. The first was one telling me that I had been awarded a 'B' merit award. This was unexpected but it essentially increased my basic salary by 50 per cent so that I could look forward to an increase of another 25 per cent over my 'C' award.

The second was from the Regional Medical Officer informing us that Geoff Whittaker was retiring and asking if any of us four programme managers was interested in taking over the Quality Assurance role on a temporary, part-time basis. I replied that I would be interested.

Priestfield was put on the market at what I thought was a highly inflated price. There were the usual few nosey parkers who came to look round but no serious offers were forthcoming near the asking price. I therefore set about raising capital to enable us to move into a smaller house. Fiona decided to stay with me, and continue to work at the General.

When out sailing in Gibraltar Bay single-handed one day, I met a single dolphin. I do not know if he was as lonely as I but he came up on my starboard quarter and started chirping away at me. I replied, out loud, that I was sorry not to be able to understand what he was saying to me. He then repeated the phrases several times in exactly the same sequence each time. I just chatted away to him about my troubles and he chirped away back for quite a long time. He then obviously got fed up with this stupid human who could not understand what he was saying and swam off. I have never had such close communication with a dolphin since.

I plucked up courage to ask Sue Sewell out for a drink one lunchtime when she had a day off. To my surprise she did not tell me to get lost but agreed to meet me in town. We got on really well and from then we quite often met at lunchtimes.

The relationship remained entirely platonic until 5 August when we were both at a Unit night out. I asked her if I could take her home and she accepted. I parked round the corner from her house and kissed her goodnight. She responded, shyly but positively. I knew at that moment I had fallen in love with her. It seems that it was mutual as we now celebrate 5 August as an additional anniversary every year. The next 18 months, however, were not to be easy for us.

In the autumn I began looking at houses and found a bungalow with a large garden and a five acre field in Oakwood, a village just outside Hexham on the north side of the Tyne valley. The house was called 'Highfield'.

Soon after finding a new house, and while waiting in the airport departure lounge to fly out to the boat, I heard an announcement, over the Tannoy, asking me to come to a phone. There was a message for me to phone 'Sue' , with a number. I assumed that this was Sue my Superintendent Radiographer with a last minute problem from the Screening Programme. I was wrong; it was Sue Sewell to wish me a good holiday. To this day neither of us know how she plucked up courage to do it. It did make my holiday though!

I had set in motion the divorce proceedings and Muriel signalled that she would not contest it. I also wanted a 'clean break' financial settlement as this had been strongly advised by the lawyer in order to avoid any claim against my income or pension at a later date.

The 30th reunion of our class from University was held in Peebles Hydro. I was embarrassed to be there on my own, for the first time, and tired of repeating the story of our separation to so many people.

In October Region informed everyone that I had agreed to take over as Quality Assurance Manager, on a part-time basis. Unfortunately this

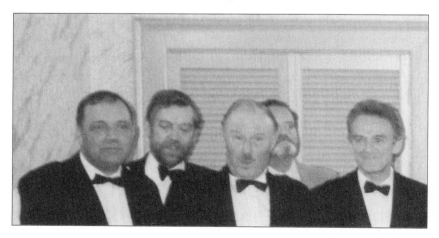

Thirty-year Class Reunion, Peebles, 1991.

took my immediate employers, the DHA and the Hospital, by surprise as I had not talked to them about it having heard nothing myself from Region since replying to their letter. A few 'rude' letters flew around but in the end it was accepted that the job would not influence my normal NHS commitments.

We had had one offer for Priestfield that was short of the sum that Muriel wanted but which I was prepared to accept to get the property off my hands. She adamantly refused and so the sale fell through and, as a result, we took it off the market for the winter. I could not, at that time, understand why she was against the offer.

Christmas and New Year were very quiet that year compared with the previous nine. The Unit night out was special in that Sue and I spent most of the evening together, which was noticed by at least one or two of her friends.

The professional bodies involved in the screening programme were all represented nationally by groups called 'Big 18s'. These consisted of representatives from each Region plus cross representation from the other specialities and a representative from the private sector. At the first meeting of the Surgeons' 'Big 18' I think there were 75 people present. I do not recall it ever falling below about 30 in the years to come owing to political in-fighting in certain parts of the country.

In early January, before we could move, Priestfield was burgled. Fiona came home just after dark and must have disturbed them. She was very shocked at the discovery but by the time I got home she had rung the police. We lost quite a few items, more of sentimental value than financial, and although some silver and ivory was stolen much was still strewn about the floors. We never recovered any of the items.

On the first weekend in February James came down from Dundee to help us move all our belongings across from Priestfield to Highfield. We did not have a dog on the property but we had found a black lurcher called Tiger. The move was slightly hindered by Tiger, who thought that he was guarding everything. We also had to introduce the two cats, Red who was a Siamese–Burmese cross and Nutty, Fiona's cat, to the new house and surroundings.

It was thus that Fiona and I, with James still in his flat in Dundee in his last year of his course, entered the last decade of the twentieth century. 1991 had been a traumatic year but it was to turn out to be a turning point in my professional and personal life.

CHAPTER EIGHTEEN

Highfield, 1992–1995

H IGHFIELD is a large 1920s bungalow with a two-room 'granny flat' in the attic which became Fiona's abode. James used the single spare room when he was down from Dundee. It was a much more practical home for us than Priestfield, was easy to run and had gas central heating.

Surrounding the house was a one-acre garden, much of it lawn, with rose beds and rhododendron bushes. To the south of the house, which overlooked the Tyne valley opposite Hexham, was a five-acre field that was used by a local farmer as the obstetric unit for his calving cows. On the north side there was a large turning circle with a new garage on one side and a 16ft by 8ft greenhouse on the other. There were one or two very old fruit trees which produced an abundance of plums and apples.

A major attraction, for me at least, was the presence of the Rat Inn which was only two fields away as the crow flies, the first being our own, but within easy walking, or staggering, distance along the country lanes.

A week after we had moved in I received my Decree Absolute from the Court. The financial settlement was to prove to be more difficult, and took another 18 months to reach final agreement.

At work there were beginning to be big changes following the introduction of the internal market in the health service. We clinicians were soon to discover that, however much the government said we were to be involved in this new management structure, it was not to happen at local level. Ever since those days clinicians have had less and less say in the organisation, and running, of the health service. We understood how the health service ran as we had been steeped in it during many years of training. It is hardly surprising that, since we were cut out, management left to outsiders, and nurses and beds whittled away, it has fallen into the depressingly poor state it is in now.

Day Case Surgery suddenly became the in thing. The current management had conveniently forgotten that the previous management had closed our five day beds as one of the first economies some years previously. We were now told that almost everything could be done as a day case.

I felt that the time was right, in the light of my taking on the Quality Assurance role, to declare myself a Breast Surgeon and cease all other cancer work while continuing to do my share of on-call and the 'bread and butter' work in general surgery.

The Breast Clinic was developing into the kind of clinic I had envisaged with one visit for most patients while we strived to get enough resources to provide a full one stop diagnostic service with instant imaging and cytology, and a dedicated in-patient unit.

I then discovered why Muriel had not wanted to sell Priestfield the previous autumn. She decided to come back north to reopen the stables as there was too much competition in the south. She made me an offer that was less than my half was worth, but I accepted to allow me to pay off my bridging loan.

I had for a long time wanted a personalised number plate and decided to treat myself to one for my 55th birthday. I managed to find RGW96X for only £250 and had the MG Turbo re-plated with that number.

The spring Moynihan Club meeting was in Lisbon in April and as I was going on my own I only went for the three days of the meeting itself. Lisbon is a lovely, if a little dusty, city and we had a good time. The president that year was Ian McLaren. He is a true Scotsman, plays the bagpipes and did so at the official dinner. I was sitting at the top table almost opposite him with a lady guest on either side. As Ian sat down after playing, he fell backwards and his chair upended with him in it on to the floor with his legs and kilt asunder. The lady on my right had an excellent view and nearly fainted.

At the Regional Office Jackie Murray took over the running of the screening programme. This was the start of a long and happy working relationship over the next few years.

James qualified BA (Hons) in Design that summer. He was not sure what he was going to do for a job but in the first instance felt that he wanted to stay in Dundee, among his friends, and look for employment there.

Sue and I were becoming even closer although the relationship was still relatively platonic. At the end of July I invited her out to see the new house and took her out to dinner at the 'General Havelock' in Haydon Bridge. This was the first time we had had dinner alone together.

It was clear that our relationship was becoming serious and that one day we were going to have to address it. It was not going to be easy as she had two children, Emma and Robbie, who were 16 and 14, as they probably would not accept Sue's relationship with me. I fully understood the situation and was prepared not to press for any immediate change.

Towards the end of the summer I felt that, as QA manager, it was time that I did a formal visit to the other three screening units in the Region. Unlike some other parts of the country we had never had formal QA visits and my arrival was viewed with suspicion by a lot of the staff.

The autumn meeting of the Moynihan Club was held in Edinburgh. It is custom for the Scottish members (by birth) to wear the kilt at the formal dinner and this is especially encouraged at the foreign meetings. I ordered a full formal set before returning home.

One Monday morning I got a phone call from the NHS Executive in London asking if I was still interested in their overseas development work. I had expressed an interest in a project to commission a surgical unit in Turkey a couple of years previously but I had been too late to get the job. I replied that I was. The person at the other end was very apologetic but said that they needed someone to go to Russia fairly soon. I replied that this was all right as I had no personal commitments. 'Soon' turned out to be that Saturday.

The major obstacle was to obtain a visa. I had to send off my passport with the knowledge that I would only see it again at Heathrow Airport at the same time as I saw the air tickets. I was confident as the person organising the trip from the NHS HQ was Douglas Hague who had previously been our Regional Chairman.

I was invited on this trip as they required the expertise of a 'surgical oncologist'. This was interesting as the term had never been accepted by the UK Colleges. The expertise was needed by a team from UK, which was designing a new Cancer Hospital in Ekaterinburg (Sverdlovsk) and they could not understand some of the requirements of the Professor in charge, Professor Tchaikovsky.

We flew to Moscow in a Boeing 757. Entry into Russia, even after the end of the cold war, was not easy. The passports and visas were checked by young soldiers through what was the old KGB central computer so one had to stand for a while waiting to see if you got the green light (literally). No one spoke to, or smiled at, these young lads and I decided to see what would happen if I did. I smiled and said, 'Good morning.' To my surprise he smiled and said, in perfect English, 'Sorry to keep you waiting, this will only take a moment.'

The next thing I discovered was that there was no toilet paper in the lavatories in the International airport. Luckily my Marine training had told me to bring a packet, together with some other vital necessities.

We were taken across Moscow where we booked in to the flight to Ekaterinburg and were handed a boarding card. 'This is new,' said one of my companions, 'first time we've had one of these.' Great, I thought, progress, until I realised that there was nothing printed on the card apart from the Aeroflot logo.

The plane was a huge Illushin troop transport. We took our own luggage out and put it in what had been the rifle rack space at the foot of a staircase up to the passenger deck. The seats were in a terrible state and many did not have any seat belt. As foreigners we had been allowed on board first and managed to find three together which all had seat belts.

It was dark by this time and we flew, at an alarmingly low level, the 1,000 miles due east to Ekaterinburg. There was no such thing as a cabin service and although there were a few stewardesses they seemed to do very little, least of all give out any safety information. I used up a year's supply of adrenalin on the two-hour trip.

It was minus 20°C when we got there and were taken in a minivan to a *dacha* in the forest outside the town. This turned out to be the one that the Tzar stayed in before he was taken away and murdered. It was a very grand building and well preserved as a guesthouse for foreign visitors and national dignitaries. There was resident staff, including a chef, and it would have been possible to ask for a meal at any time of day or night.

The next morning it had snowed some more. We were picked up by the minivan and taken into town to the offices of the British Health Care Consortium to meet the Professor. There was a certain air of the KGB about the place and true enough, the chief had been a KGB Colonel and his secretary a female KGB Major. We discovered that when the regime collapsed the KGB members got most of the good jobs in tourism and commerce.

Professor Tchaikovsky and I hit it off immediately even though he could speak no English, and I no Russian. The problem I was there to solve related to the flow of patients from a ward, through the operating theatre and into recovery. He had one idea and the architect another. The Russians had not seen the modern theatre design: in through an anaesthetic room and out through a recovery room. We agreed within an hour that we could work together and solve it.

To do this he invited us back to his hospital to see his own plans. These turned out to be in the form of a three dimensional, computer graphic, rotating diagram of the surgical block with cartoon figures moving a trolley from the ward to, and through, the operating theatre. I then described how we would suggest changing the routing slightly and I had done my job within two hours of starting it.

They took me next to see their operating theatres. The main theatre was not a twin one, as we are used to, but a triple one. This, also unlike ours, was not divided into separate rooms but there were three operating tables in the one room with three operations going on at once. One had just finished and the patient was taken away on a trolley. The next patient was walked in straight to the operating table in the middle, and invited to climb up on to it. She was then left alone for a few minutes until the anaesthetist returned from waking up her predecessor.

That evening the Russians laid on a banquet at the *dacha*. There were four glasses of various sizes at each place. These were for vodka, wine, beer and water in ascending size. We were told that the best way to

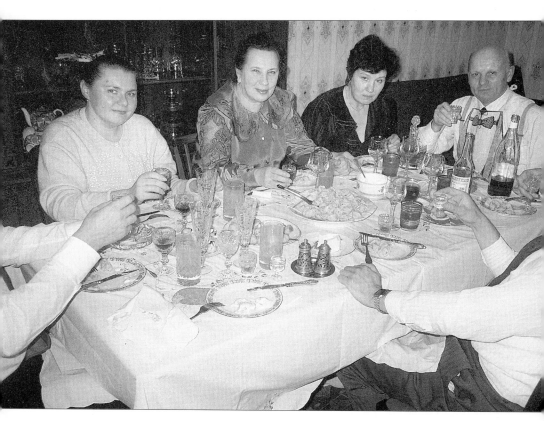

Professor Tchaikovsky's dinner party, Ekaterinburg, 1992.

'survive' one of these sessions was to drink one of each of these drinks as a set. It was indeed to prove to be a session as they have a tradition that for every speech there has to be a reply and after every speech a glass of vodka is downed in one. As there were eight people present and the session did not start till after the two National toasts we had a great deal to drink. The following day we did not have hangovers.

We went to the Government building for the Urals, to meet the Minister of Finance. He was a bluff and fairly bluntly rude man called Nosov. We were there to try to get his agreement to spending the money to build this hospital. Mr Nosov eventually nodded gravely, and agreed that the project should go ahead.

That night Professor Tchaikovsky invited us round to his 'house' to meet his family and some friends. I say 'house' as he lived in one of the huge blocks of flats that almost everyone seemed to live in there. He had a tiny, two bedroom, flat in which he, his wife, and one of his sons and his wife and child, all lived. His annual salary was about the same as one month's of mine. We arrived to find everyone who lived in the block seemed to be out on the stairs to see and greet us. They had never seen, let alone met, anyone from the West.

Very early the next morning I had to catch the 'business flight', alone, back to Moscow. It was minus 21°C and I expected them to de-ice the aircraft before leaving. The plane was a Tu 154, similar but smaller than the three-engine Boeing 727. It was only in slightly better state than the one on the way there. They did have newspapers (Russian) and steward-esses but still no safety instructions.

We took off without de-icing, shuddering our way down the runway and staggering off the ground. It was just daylight by this stage and the whole countryside was covered in snow. Two hours later we approached Moscow and a blizzard started as we descended. I could see nothing at all, except large snowflakes, until the plane had actually touched down.

I was met by a couple in a small Lada taxi. The driver was a Jewish violin player who was waiting for permission to emigrate to the West. His wife was a teacher and he dropped us in Moscow to sightsee before taking me to the airport. I wanted to get a feel for the place and the people so we went down to the Arbat shopping and street-market area. Things were obviously in short supply but, contrary to TV programmes made at that time, there was coffee and vodka readily available in the shops, at a price.

Leaving the country you have to declare your possessions to a customs man who x-rays the cases and stamps a form. As he stamped my form I said, 'Thank you.' He paused, looked at me and smiled. Again in

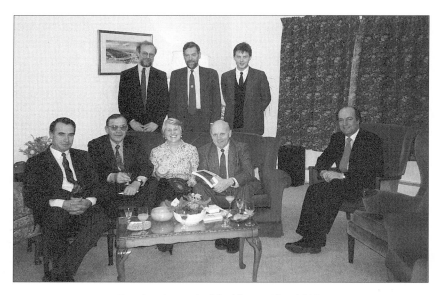

Russian 'return' visit, Newcastle, 1993.

perfect English he said, 'I hope you have enjoyed your stay in Russia, Mr Wilson.' I may have made his day and he certainly made mine as I gratefully boarded the BA 757 for the flight back to London.

On my return I attended the first of the National QA Managers' meeting in London at the beginning of December and found that, like the Evaluation group, I was working with people who were dedicated to the screening programme and who understood it in depth.

The surgical unit Christmas night out was held on 22 December when Sue and I spent most of the evening together. It was about this time that Sue's off-duty started to appear in my diary. There was little doubt that it was not a question of whether we would get together but simply when. She was, not surprisingly, worried about her children and how they would react and cope with any such dramatic event.

One of the places that I had always wanted to visit was Madeira. I went there at the end of January where I found a lovely 'British' summer climate and a rather old world Portuguese culture. I had a thoroughly good time there although I would have preferred to have Sue with me.

Professor Tchaikovsky wanted to pay a return visit to see for himself some of the things we had told him about. He arrived in Newcastle on 24 February and visited the Radiotherapy and Oncology Unit at the General, and the new operating theatres at Freeman Hospital.

I could see that Sue was close to making a decision to come and live with me and we started to look at Highfield from this point of view. There being insufficient wardrobe space for a full set of lady's clothes we ordered a complete set of bedroom furniture from MFI which rather committed us to us getting together.

One weekend in early March she helped me build the wardrobes, chest of drawers etc and this left her with the agonising decision as to how and when to break the news to all her family. In the event it happened suddenly on Thursday 27 March when she arrived with her belongings in black plastic bags. It was a traumatic time for Sue particularly, leaving her children, as they would not come with her and she desperately wanted them to. We both worried equally about how her parents would react and cope, as they are of a generation not used to such happenings. Apart from Sandra, Sue's best friend, the only ones who knew in advance were Sue's sister Elaine, my daughter Fiona, and Ken Queen who had been such a good friend and confident the year before.

I had to register her with my GP, Steve Ford, at Haydon Bridge. I took her over to introduce her and he caused some consternation, and not a little amusement, by asking what contraception we were using. Neither Sue nor I had given it a moment's thought. I suppose he was absolutely right to ask.

I was very keen to introduce Sue to my part of Spain, and Duquesa in particular, and rented an apartment in the port. I was pleased that Sue liked it although she was not keen on sailing unless the sea was flat calm.

The Moynihan Club was due to hold the next meeting in Malta at the beginning of May. I had decided that I would not give the secretary a chance to prevent me taking Sue so I simply booked her in with me. Everyone was very nice to her, and I wore my new kilt for the very first time in public at the dinner.

On our return I resolved to try to give Sue as much security as was possible without actually being married. I went to see John Luke, my family lawyer, and we constructed a rather complicated will in Sue's favour, without leaving out my children. He also told me that there was no law against being engaged to someone who was still married. I looked out my mother's engagement ring and 'popped the question' one evening. I am pleased to say she accepted and we became formally engaged. To get over the problem that she couldn't officially become a 'Wilson' we had notepaper and cards printed that said 'Sue and Ron Wilson'.

I had resolved to buy Sue a new car and get her a personalised number plate to coincide with 1 August 1993. I managed to get her L5 SJW, having just missed L4 SJW by one day. We chose a pillar-box red Rover 220si coupé and, although not quite as powerful as the MG Turbo, it went very fast.

The autumn meeting of the Moynihan club was held in Newcastle. It was only Sue's second meeting with the Club and was obviously quite a challenge for her, but most things went smoothly and I was very pleased that she was getting on well with the other wives. The question still on people's lips, however, was, 'When are you getting married?'

All efforts to preserve the General Hospital had just failed following a meeting held at Seaham to thrash out the future of hospital services in Newcastle and the preferred option of Region's which was to make the General into a Community Hospital was accepted.

At the same time as we were getting this depressing news the QA Guidelines for Surgeons in Breast Cancer Screening was published as an official Screening Programme publication. Included in the document were the proformas we had developed to record the treatment and follow-up on the computer system.

Nosov, from Ekaterinburg, came to Newcastle in mid-October, and we showed him round but this time our Managers failed to show up at the lunch that had been arranged for him to meet people. Considering that he was the equivalent of our Chancellor of the Exchequer, in the Urals, I felt that this was something of a blunder.

Douglas Hague and I had debated as to how to entertain him; as I had been to Professor Tchaikovsky's house it was suggested that he come to mine. All this was decided the day before he was due and left poor Sue with little time to organise any supper. To give her more time on her own to prepare the supper Douglas and I took him, and his interpreter, to the Rat. The fire was lit as it was beginning to be cold at nights and Nosov really loved the atmosphere, never having been in an English pub before. We had to drag him away in the end before the supper was ruined. We had a thoroughly good evening at Highfield and my idea that he was a boorish, old style, Russian Communist were completely shattered.

In the nine months since Sue and I had been together I still had not met Steve and Jean, her mother and father; nor, officially, her sister Elaine and her husband Pete. We arranged to meet at the Lion and Lamb, a restaurant half way between Newcastle and Hexham. The evening went smoothly and we all got on well. Steve and Jean then came for Christmas lunch with Fiona and James.

I had for some months been calculating my pension entitlement and had been in touch with Lytham St Anne's to get confirmation of its value. I calculated that I could retire at 61 and really did not want to contemplate carrying on any longer. A question uppermost in my mind was where to retire to? I was torn between Duquesa and my latest find: Madeira.

I had wanted to introduce Sue to the island since I had visited the island the year before. On this trip, in January 1994, we stayed at the Quinta del Sol, a family hotel opposite the rather posh Savoy that I had stayed in on the previous trip. It was a comfortable walk into Funchal although on the way back it is uphill. This was to prove a real problem on one occasion when we had been to one of the Madeira wine tasting sessions in the town and consumed a large quantity of the product. We were staggering up the hill when I caught my spectacle loops in a hedge.

James was offered a job by John Dodd, Johnathan's father, in his GRP factory. He moved to live with Johnathan and another friend, in Jesmond in Newcastle. He moved his 'heirloom piano' from Highfield to Jesmond.

My professional life was now almost entirely taken up with Breast Cancer and Screening. I was spending a lot of time on QA work in the Region as well as with the National Committees I was on. I would during this year spend up to two days a week travelling to London and other cities for meetings.

In April the Acute services at the General came under the control of the RVI Trust and we, the staff, with it. We had no say in the matter and our contracts were simply moved. Radiotherapy, on the General site, came under the control of Freeman Hospital as did their buildings and equipment. The buildings that housed us were to be under the control of a new, third Trust, the City Health Trust, thus making life very, and unnecessarily, complicated for everybody. The new trust was essentially an amalgamation of the Mental Health services, and the new Community Health ideas that were in vogue.

Ken Queen and his wife sadly split up and Ken left Shotley Bridge to take up a pure Urology post in Dunfermline in Scotland. I was still examining in Edinburgh three times a year and arranged to meet him there for dinner as it is not far over the Forth to Dunfermline. He had settled into the new job but was having a difficult time over the divorce and had not yet managed to find a home for himself up there.

At the end of April the Moynihan Club meeting was held in Vienna. This was a new city to both Sue and me and we had a thoroughly good time indeed. We saw the Vienna Boys' Choir, the Spanish Riding School and several famous palaces. It is very expensive indeed.

I think it was about this time that I came to the conclusion that

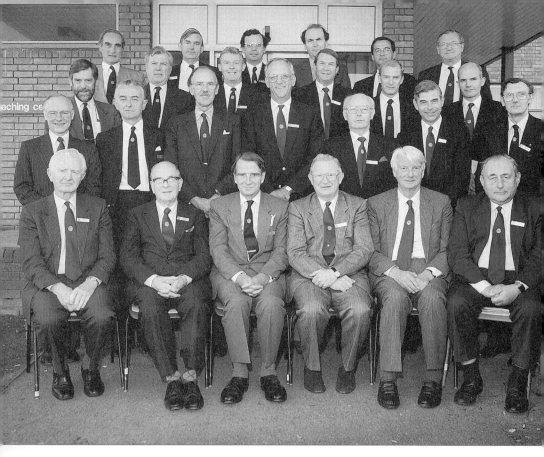

Moynihan Club meeting, Newcastle, 1993.

things in the NHS were never going to be as they had been. There were new changes in the junior staff allocation, tied up with the new 'Calman' training programme that, for the first time, was abandoning the apprenticeship type of training. It was envisaged by some people, who should have known better, that all routine and emergency work would be done by Consultants. This would have needed a doubling of our numbers as the number of 'hands on' juniors dropped. This increase did not happen, as many of us predicted, and Consultants found themselves working even harder than before.

I went to Gibraltar in July where I was joined by Sue after the first week but her suitcase failed to arrive, We got her suitcase the following night but realised that it had been opened and searched. What had interested the customs was a small bag of white powder that Sue always took on holiday with her together with some teabags. The fact that the white powder was sugar would not have become apparent to the customs until they had opened it.

We were definitely apartment, or house, hunting and heard of a house in a typically Andalucían Urbanisation about two miles from the port. It belonged to a 70 year old former Spitfire pilot who wanted to go back to England and into sheltered accommodation. We fell in love with the house at the first visit. It is a two-bedroomed, open plan house almost completely surrounded by a small, but lovely, garden. The views over the sea and back towards Gibraltar are breathtaking. We inherited two tortoises although at that time of year they are hard to find in the vegetation. They were both the same size and could usually be found by the noise of their sexual activities that were quite enthusiastic. We hoped we had inherited a male and a female.

Fiona, who initially had planned to live with Mark prior to getting married, had changed her mind and they decided to get married at the end of August. I was not happy about the match but as in so many cases these days there is not a lot a parent can say, or do, to dissuade their offspring.

The week before the wedding we had a rehearsal followed by a meal for both families at the Raven Hotel where the reception was to be held. This was the first time I had seen Muriel since she had left and I found it difficult, with John present, but not as bad as I had feared. I had to go to Priestfield on the morning of the wedding to pick up Fiona so that she could leave from there. This I found much worse as it used to be my home.

It seemed an anathema to me that the Breast and Cervical Screening Programmes should be run completely separately and, although there was a National QA scheme in breast, there was no such monitoring in cervical. The Northern Region started to bring to the two programmes closer together and I, as the QA Manager albeit part time, began to be invited to the Regional steering group meetings of the latter programme.

The use of treatment protocols, and proper data recording of the treatment, in the screening programme was beginning to expand across the country and as one of the first proponents of this found myself being invited to other Regions to talk on the subject and to try to persuade people to use the computer programme we had provided. This then led me to be invited on to the Computer Development Team, for the Programme, which plans the continued upgrading of the system year by year.

The rest of the year was pretty hectic with continued frequent trips to London and many local and Regional meetings. One of the new topics for discussion was the place of genetics particularly in breast cancer as it had become possible to screen for two of the genes. Only about 5 to 10 per cent of all cases at the most were genetically linked and I was concerned that too much emphasis was beginning to be placed on family history. This led to most breast clinics having to develop a protocol with their local genetics department, to cope with this new demand from the public, but there was never any official funding for it.

The New Year party, in Spain, was held in three houses in succession. It started in our house with drinks and nibbles, moved next door for a buffet supper and then on next door again for the actual New Year. In Spain the 'ex-pats' celebrate two separate new years, one hour apart. The first is typically Spanish with fresh grapes (12: one for each hour chimed and eaten with each chime) and champagne and the second typically British, very alcoholic.

At about 2 to 2.30 a.m. we set off for home, at least 150 yards away down a slight slope. Half way I fell over and as it was quite warm and I was quite comfortable lying on the grass I decided to stay there. Luckily Sue decided otherwise and got me home. I had, not surprisingly, a serious hangover the next morning.

The Combined Breast Clinic on Tuesday mornings was getting so busy that I had to convert my Thursday Clinic into an overflow for the large number of new cases. We were seeing all ladies within two weeks of their referral and it was important to give them reassurance with a single visit wherever possible. For many thousands of ladies this had been the case since 1977. Only one, who was squeezed into a Thursday clinic so that she could be seen quickly, ever complained and that was only after cancer was diagnosed some years later.

In the middle of March I had a number of meetings in London. One was the surgical '18+', as I had come to call it, which was chaired as usual by Roger Blamey. I was there as the surgical representative of the Northern Region but as Julietta Patnick, the National Co-ordinator, had given her apologies was also the only representative of the National Programme present.

I felt that Roger was taking too many decisions without the agreement of Julietta and on a couple of occasions pointed this out to him. He was not pleased at my intervention of behalf of the Programme and the meeting got very tense indeed. Julietta arrived at lunchtime, I told her of the morning's happenings and at the beginning of the afternoon session she made a number of cogent remarks to Roger, about his funding in particular. The day ended on a very unhappy and unpleasant note and on the train home, maybe for the very first time, I felt very stressed.

Friday 24 March 1995 began like any other Friday with the Surgical Unit's X-ray conference in the X-ray department at 9 a.m. After this I would, normally, do a ward round and then teach the 4th year medical students. As I went towards the wards I began to have one of my attacks of 'bronchospasm' and, my inhaler being in my jacket pocket upstairs in my office, decided to go upstairs and have a 'puff'.

I remember getting half way up the stairs and then no more until I woke up in a hospital bed with Sue holding my right hand. She was telling me that I had had a heart attack but that 'I was all right now'. As I gradually rejoined the world I realised I was in the Coronary Care Unit at the General, that I was attached to an ECG monitor and had a drip in my left arm. I also noticed that my arms were totally black and blue. The time was 3 p.m. and Sue told me it was Saturday.

I had been found on the floor of the landing outside my office and Ward 20. The first year nurse who had found me had had hysterics after she raised the alarm but thanks to her quick thinking Mike Griffin was quickly on the scene followed by Rob Bullock, the Anaesthetist. Between them, with advice from Keith Evemy the Cardiologist, they had made my chest black and blue during two hours of resuscitating me 'from a cardiac arrest' on the landing floor. They had also used the defibrillator on me as I was in Ventricular Fibrillation and I had superficial burns to prove it.

I felt physically drained and slightly puzzled as I had had no chest pain and had apparently got into my office and back out again as I was found clutching the inhaler in my hand.

After a week in CCU I was entrusted to Sue who took me home to Highfield. I was happy and relieved to be home but almost immediately the psychological impact of what had happened to me began to affect me. I started to have bad dreams and was afraid to go to sleep, fearing that I would not wake up again. Finally I began to have panic attacks (as I called them) in the middle of the night with anxiety, sweating and palpitations. On 4 April I had such a bad attack that we called the doctor who, not wishing to take any risks, bundled me straight into Hexham General Hospital.

After monitoring me for 48 hours and checking my enzymes, I was allowed home again after consultations with Keith.

My immediate need was for relaxation therapy that I learned from a book and a tape provided by the District Nurse. In this one you are encouraged to think of a beautiful house with a flowing staircase, lovely furniture and garden outside. I changed that to thinking of naughty thoughts about Sue; it worked a charm and I began to sleep much better.

A month later I had to go back to the General for the first of my exercise tests – 'The Treadmill'. I believe that if you can survive the full test, to the level required of you, you will survive almost anything, in the short term at least.

I returned to part-time work in mid June, just under three months from my arrest. It had been agreed that at first I would only do outpatient clinics, a little teaching and administration with a Senior Registrar, who was very experienced, covering my nights on call with me nominally the Consultant on call. In the event of any major trauma my colleagues arranged to be available to help the Senior Registrar.

My physical recovery was remarkably quick. Not so my psychological one. For years I had wondered if I would reach the age my father died at 48, and then the age that my mother died at 54, both of them from myocardial infarctions. I had been 58 on 20 April, four weeks after mine, and I could not shake off the niggling thought that I had survived this one but what about the next one, and when would it happen?

At the General another ward was closed and turned into a Day Surgery Unit. It was becoming clear that transfer to the RVI was inevitable. We were, however, expected to continue the same level of service with only two wards instead of four, and with fewer junior staff, the remainder of whom were working to strict new hours limitations under the 'New Deal'.

Consultants found their workload and stress levels rising. We were asked to write a job plan. This produced a conservative estimate of 49 hours a week for routine clinical work that did not include my managerial work for the Programme and the Region. In addition I was contractually supposed to be on call one night in four from 5 p.m. to 8 a.m. the next morning. Any of the junior doctors who now worked these hours automatically had the next day off.

My attempts to return to full-time working showed up not only physical weakness but that my confidence had really taken a knock; worse than at first apparent. I became tense during operating and for the first time in my career began to doubt if decisions had been the correct ones. Even the simplest of operations would cause stress and during one emergency procedure I had a panic attack.

I had also stopped wanting to take the boat out when we were in Spain and since I had sailed all my life since the age of fourteen realised that this was a significant problem. After a few weeks it was obvious that I could not go on like this either for the benefit to my patients' health, or my own. I confided in Malcolm Clague, who was by now the Clinical Director of Surgery for the whole Trust, that I was not coping and that I felt I would have to revert to part-time. He accepted my feelings but suggested that I had to tell Occupational Health.

This I did and was gratified when, after 'plucking up courage' to admit my problem, they said that this was not unusual and that maybe I had gone back to work too early. They referred me, with my consent of course, to a Clinical Psychologist.

I went to the first appointment in fear and trepidation as I, like most senior doctors, had never had to seek such advice and help before. Dr Wilkinson was charming and put me at ease immediately; we talked through the problem and possible ways to improve things. I got some of my confidence back but I came to realise that it was unlikely that I would ever be able to fully fulfil my role as a full-time consultant general surgeon again.

Sue and I had decided that Highfield was too much for us, under the circumstances, and to find a smaller home. We sold the cars but retained our number plates and bought a matching pair of Fiat Cinquecentos, black and canary yellow.

We started to search for a new home and decided that we both wanted to stay in the Corbridge/Hexham area. We sold Highfield and, armed with cash and no need for a mortgage, came across a 1960s bungalow at the end of a cul-de-sac. It was on the other side of the Tyne Valley directly opposite Oakwood, at the eastern end of Hexham.

My opposite number QA manager in the Yorkshire Region left for another job. Northern and Yorkshire were now one and in order to allow discussion as to how to proceed in QA I was asked if I would support the Yorkshire end as well, while a review of the provision of the service was undertaken. I agreed but stressed that it could only be temporarily and that they, at Region, would have to clear it with my long suffering employer.

A remaining concern was what was to become of Tiger who was not a town dog. Red, the cat, would be no problem and there was a cat door there already. In the end the new owners of Highfield, who had had cats but never a dog, offered to keep him at Highfield. We were delighted and indeed they spoiled him even more than we did and we heard that he soon became a housedog.

Now that we had found our smaller home I felt the time had come to prepare the ground for taking early retirement. I again calculated my pension and based on my 'B' award I had enough years in to retire after I was 61, two years away. I was certain that I would not be able to fulfil my job commitment till than and I also was sure the Trust would not let me work part-time for ever. I therefore wrote to them suggesting that I retire, on grounds of ill health, after my next birthday in April 1996, when I would be 59, and asking to discuss possible terms.

I was a little hamstrung because Sue and I were not yet married and therefore she could not inherit any pension if I retired before we could get married, or if I died in the meantime. A further complication was the recent introduction of five-yearly reviews on the merit awards, which in itself I support, but mine was on-going and due to be extended, or otherwise, in the spring of 1996. The timing was not auspicious.

I began to visit the Yorkshire QA Offices on a regular basis where Carol Candler, who had been part of my team in Newcastle, was the co-ordinator. The office was based at Cookridge Hospital, Leeds, which is on the western outskirts but can be approached from the north via Harrogate and took about two hours in good traffic. I then had to start visiting the four screening Units in Leeds itself, York, Hull and Bradford. Their QA and Operational procedures were different from ours but not so as to cause me a problem. I did think, however, that their QA was a lot more lax than in the north, even though we had never done formal QA visits or inspections.

We were now ready to move and while I had loved Highfield I realised that it was too big for us both now. It had not been Sue's choice of house whereas our new one in Spain, and now this one in Hexham, was to be ours rather than mine.

CHAPTER NINETEEN

Hexham and Spain, 1996–1998, and Retirement

W<small>E MOVED</small> across the Tyne valley on 8 January 1996 and Sue obtained her Decree Nisi later in the month. We began to plan our wedding for immediately after the six week waiting period would be up and took a bit of a gamble by setting a date of 29 March without the Decree Absolute. We settled for a Registry Office wedding in Hexham, with only close family as guests.

Region had decided that they wanted one QA manager for the whole of the new Northern and Yorkshire area and that he/she would be responsible for both the Breast and the Cervical Programmes. This was in line with a subsequent decision by the Department of Health for the National Programmes. Jackie Murray asked me if I would be interested in the post and I replied that I could only do it if I could first retire from my current post.

I had two meetings with Peter Hill, the Deputy Director of Public Health, and a more formal interview, with the Personnel Officer present, when we came to the agreement that I would take on the role for a two-year, part-time contract as soon as I retired.

Sue's Decree Absolute came through on 12 March. After three years of waiting we were able to get married at last. I found the civil ceremony much better than a religious one. In the evening we had booked the restaurant, at the Angel in Corbridge for a buffet and a disco for forty of our other friends. Ken came up from Cardiff with Jen, his new partner whom he had known for a long time and whom he was soon to marry. David and Lynne Deacon, whom I hadn't seen for many years, came up and both couples stayed at the Angel which is just as well as they consumed a lot of drink.

At one stage Sue was dancing on a door table top with Dr Dave Moor. I took a couple of photographs, which was just as well because

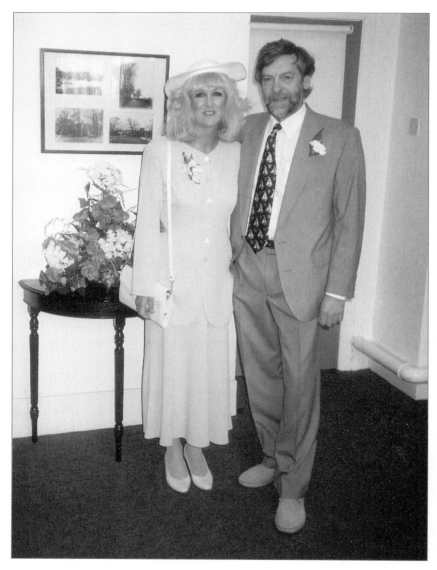

Our wedding, 1996.

most people afterwards couldn't remember, or believe, that she had done it. We honeymooned in Paris.

I was relieved that all had worked out especially for Sue. We had to go through a second rigmarole of changing her passport and credit cards and arrange yet another pair of wills plus one in Spain as their inheritance laws are different to ours.

I wrote officially to the Trust proposing that I should retire at the end of June on the grounds that I could not fulfil all my contractual obligations as a Consultant Surgeon, thus giving them the required three months' formal notice. This was accepted and I started with Region a week later.

All this was at the height of the purchaser-provider phase of the health service and I had a strange arrangement whereby I was acting for Region but was employed by the City Health Trust, who employed all the rest of the staff, and where the office was based. I was, however, responsible to the purchaser of the service who was based in Leeds.

Sue's daughter Emma had gone to Tenerife to work, having found her office job in the Northern Rock boring and Sue, with her mother, went to stay out there for a week in May. Although she came home for a short time Emma spent nearly three years out there altogether.

One of my last administrative tasks in my role of junior trainee tutor and adviser to the College of Surgeons, was to host an official inspection visit by a College team. I had always held the view that if the acute services were to be moved off the General site it would have to be a total move. This was not wholly achieved by the current plan in that Trauma, Neurosurgery and Radiotherapy were remaining on the site that was soon to be without surgical support. Three sites working for any speciality was not really an option any more and the College rules, if I recalled them correctly, meant this was not an acceptable arrangement for training purposes.

I, and the two College Assessors, tried to point this out particularly as it related to Trauma/Orthopaedic training but maybe also for general surgery, and that accreditation of some posts might be in jeopardy. The assessors produced a damning report that upset almost everyone at the RVI, the Freeman, our Trust and the University. I was personally accused of failing to notify some of the 'key players' about the meeting and I received several very rude and angry letters. I sent back copies of minutes of meetings where I had reminded everyone of the importance of this visit and that they should make every effort to let their junior staff attend, and to attend themselves.

It gave me the greatest pleasure, however, to send two of the most vociferous and senior critics copies of their own letters declining to meet the team. I could not wait to get out of such antagonistic politics that were ruining a perfectly good service in the City. I understand that the problems have rumbled on ever since.

I retired from all clinical practice at the end of June 1996. I had decided that it was only correct that if I was not fit to continue my job it was not appropriate to do any clinical work whatsoever. This not only saved on all the various professional expenses but in particular I did not have to continue to pay to be insured. I have never regretted this complete break.

The screening unit, the outpatients, the wards and theatres all gave leaving parties for me. I was presented with a set of matching luggage and a box of personal momentos from the theatre staff. My surgical colleagues had arranged a whole day symposium, in the teaching centre at the General, which was a mixture of science and good fun. In the evening they had arranged a private dinner party in the Fisherman's Lodge for only my closest friends and it was a very memorable evening.

After 19 years in the post at the General I found it sad and emotional but I was relieved to be going under the circumstances, especially since the General was about to lose its identity. I treated myself to a new MGF sports car with some of my lump sum. I say 'myself' as it has Sue's number on it and she refers to it as 'her car'.

The new job presented me with two main challenges, later to be increased to three. The first was to integrate the eight breast screening units into a single Northern and Yorkshire environment and introduce a single, uniform, QA system. The second was to develop a parallel QA system for the new enlarged Region for the Cervical Screening programme. Both were to encounter considerable resistance; the former from the Yorkshire teams who resented what they saw as a Northern takeover, and the latter from almost everyone in the cervical programme who resented a 'breast man' telling them what to do.

We had not completed the work when it was decided, at National level, that QA visits (inspections) were to be introduced. I knew my own four units well enough to know that there was unlikely to be a problem unearthed by such a visit that I did not know about already. I had serious doubts about two of the programmes in Yorkshire, mainly due to the autocracy of the Programme Managers and the previous lax QA control over their work practices.

To tackle the cervical screening QA we formed a Regional working party of five to draw up proposals as how to approach the completely different problems associated with that programme. We appointed Marion, a very experienced nurse with knowledge of the community, two 'Bills' – the first from the Yorkshire end with an existing reputation at National level in Cytology and the second an IT expert who had previously worked for the Regional Office, and Gillian who was the administrator cum secretary whose job was also to keep me right. Now with two parallel sets of committees my life was fairly hectic and involved quite a bit of travelling holding meetings at venues that suited most people.

Early in the New Year we were asked if we, in the Northern and Yorkshire Regions, would like to participate in a screening trial of the over 65s. The idea had originated in Wakefield and was immediately supported by Age Concern, although they really wanted to go for immediate screening of all over 65s. This would have been impossible as it would require an increase in resources of one third nationally.

In meetings with all the disciplines involved I, from the outset, tried to make it clear that they would be the people advising us on how to do it and we were only the overseeing body for the Region.

At the Project Board meetings of the Programmes, which essentially used the same computer system, it was clear to all that what was really required was a totally new system. The current one had been designed to accept and store information, which it was good at. What was needed, however, was a system that could also give information back to the users so that we could continually assess the efficacy of the programmes.

The pan-Regional QA committee of the breast screening programme agreed a draft set of guidelines for formal QA visits based on National targets and guidelines. The cervical screening working party had also produced its first report and we presented our proposals for a Regional QA structure. This was based directly on our experience in the breast programme. The team then set off round all the District co-ordinating groups to explain our proposals.

It was a difficult decision but we sold *Murella*. In spite of being retired I never recovered my confidence to take her out in anything but the calmest days. It was becoming an expensive exercise just to keep her in good condition and the next time the insurance was due I was going to have to pay for a full survey. She went firstly to a teacher in Gibraltar but it was not really the right sort of boat for him and then to Guntar, a German who likes to sail her single-handed like I did.

The QA visits revealed that there was a problem in the Humberside Unit of under diagnosis in the first screen. It was not easy to get to the bottom of the problem as not only had the programme manager retired, but one of the other important members of staff had moved out of the area. I reported my concerns to Professor Donaldson and he instructed me to carry out a review of their films.

The review was entirely confidential but the 'big brother' fear was causing us continued trouble in our attempts to make progress with the cervical QA plans. I was encountering a lot of opposition from both the pathologists and the GPs. This latter group has a completely different contract of service to the rest of the professionals involved and many felt disinclined to be monitored, or told how to do things, by someone else.

A film reading failure also occurred in Exeter. In that case the QA team had made previous comments that had been ignored but which might have prevented it reaching proportions that made national headlines. The 'Exeter incident' led the Department of Health to set up a working party to review the QA process, responsibilities and funding in the breast screening programme. I was asked to give evidence to the committee.

Sue and I had a number of 'would like to dos'. One of these was to fly on Concorde and another was to travel on the Orient Express. For some months I had been secretly planning a trip that involved flying Concorde to Venice, another of Sue's 'must visit's, staying on the Lido in the Excelsior, where Churchill used to go to paint, and returning by the Orient Express via Paris. I also arranged for us to go to Florence, for a day, by train. I managed to keep this a secret from Sue until the morning we were due to fly from Heathrow.

The majority of the hard work in planning the cervical QA system was completed and only needed agreement from the disciplines involved which continued to be a slow uphill mission. At National level our proposals had met with approval and the team, who had done most of the hard work, presented our plan to their opposite numbers from across the country.

I was beginning to realise that I was again suffering from stress and working many more hours a week than my contract. I took the decision to retire from the job early, at the end of March and the NHS year. Everything I had set out to do would be finished by then so there seemed no need to stay on another three months when a new Manager could take over at this time.

Early in 1998 Region had to advertise for, and appoint, someone to succeed me. I had someone in mind but of course the post now had got to go to open competition. I was delighted when the panel decided that 'my candidate' was the best choice, on the day, and offered him the job.

Not such good news for me was that, in the reorganisation of the Trusts in Newcastle, there had been a decision taken to move the screening and assessment service, and the screening office, to the RVI. This had all been decided without reference to any of us at Region who were in a position to agree or disagree with the decision. I was sorry to see this happen as it meant the end of plans to have all the breast work at the General. It also meant that all the work was going to be done in much less spacious surroundings.

I complained that the Programme should have been consulted about any such move but realised that it was more or less a *fait-accompli* and as I would no longer be involved felt that people having made their own beds they would have to lie on them. The new unit opened in the RVI on 12 March 1998.

On the 20th there was a farewell gathering for me at Region where I was presented with a port decanter. I suspected Sue's hand in this again, as I didn't have one. Professor Donaldson, who we tipped (correctly) to get the Chief Medical Officer's post after Kenneth Calman, had asked me on a couple of occasions in the previous weeks if I wasn't going to be bored doing nothing. I had decided quite firmly in my mind that I was going to retire completely this time and declined to consider doing anything except enjoy myself.

The staff at the Reference Centre had a private farewell the day before I officially left and presented me with a Terry Wogan TOG sweater that I wear a lot, and a small Mr Blobby. They knew that both of those characters caused me mirth. I left the office finally on Friday 27 March 1998, a month short of my deadline of my 61st birthday, and nearly 42 years after I had gone to Medical School.

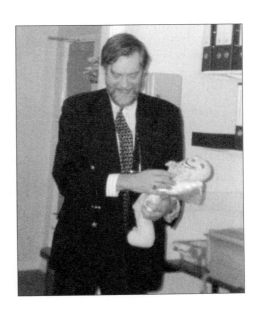

Retirement, 1998.

Postscript

OUR FOUR CHILDREN are grown up now:
James, the eldest, has moved to Edinburgh and works for a Design Consultancy that was responsible for the restoration of RY *Britannia*. He lives in a farm cottage with his Dutch fiancée – Kirsten.

Fiona, as predicted, separated from Mark after four years. She has bought a small house in Newcastle, still works in the Works Department Office, and is enjoying being reunited with all her old friends.

Emma, who enjoys working with people, is a ground hostess at Newcastle Airport with Servisair. She has also bought a small house in Newcastle.

Robbie, the youngest, is doing well in the retail car trade and has his own flat in Fenham, Newcastle.

Since retiring Sue and I have spent a lot of time at our house in Spain but have also travelled widely with the Moynihan Chirurgical Club, as well as on our own.

The only offspring of our own are an increasing number of baby tortoises in Spain.

At the end of August 2000 we went to the Far East. I wanted to show Sue that part of the world, Singapore, Sarawak and Sabah, where I had spent over two years 35 years ago. I also wanted to visit Mother's grave which I had not seen since she had been moved from Ulu Pandan cemetery to the Commonwealth War Graves Memorial Cemetery at Kranji.

The Cemetery is in the north of the island and on the day we intended to visit I phoned in advance saying we were coming to see Mother's grave. We were met by a delightful Chinese Malay, Mr Lee, who found her grave for us and led us to it. It is in a lovely spot, on a gentle slope surrounded by trees. Her grave was well tended with a little plant in front of it. What was really sad was that she was almost completely surrounded by children aged from a few days to a few years. I thought how happy she would be to be among children and left telling her 'to look after them'.

I have always been sorry that she did not live to see what I made of the career for which she sacrificed so much to launch her 'medical man'. I hope she would have approved and felt that all her hard work had not been in vain.

Index